MW01502673

For Perry,

Best Wishes for the
New Year.

Love,

Lois —

A Glow In The Dark

Lois Samuels

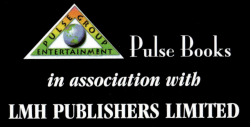

Pulse Books

in association with

LMH PUBLISHERS LIMITED

© 1999, Lois Samuels
First Edition 1999
10 9 8 7 6 5 4 3 2 1

All rights reserved. No part of this book may be reproduced, stored in a retrieval system, or transmitted, in any form or by any means, eletronic, mechanical, photocopying, recording, or otherwise, without the prior written permission of the publishers or author.

The publishers have made every effort to trace the copyright holders but if they have inadvertently overlooked any, they will be pleased to make the necessary arrangements at the first opportunity.

If you have bought this book without a cover you should be aware that it is "stolen" property. The publishers/author have not received any payment for the "stripped" book, if it is printed without their authorization.

Publishing concept: Mike Henry, LMH Publishers Limited.
Text edited by: Julia Tan (Singapore)
Text design/layout: Julia-Mei Tan (Singapore)
Arlene Schleifer Goldberg (New York)
Typeset in Garamond.
Typeset by: Michelle Mitchell (Jamaica)

Published by: LMH Publishers Limited.
7 Norman Road,
LOJ Industrial Complex
Building 10
Kingston C.S.O., Jamaica
Email Address: henryles@cwjamaica.com

ISBN 976-610-157-4 (P)
ISBN 976-610-180-9 (C)

Printed in China

For my love, Alexander Kaletski for helping me to strike the match.

Acknowledgements

My thanks to:
Dad, Mom, Judine, Aunt Adassa
Kingsley Cooper, Linda Biggs-Peart, Marsha-Marie Samuels, Tanya Russell,
Michael Charles, Christoph Reucker, John Moore,
Bethann Hardison, Tyronne Barrington, LMH Publishers Limited
David Gordon and Mr. Louis Russell who passed on.

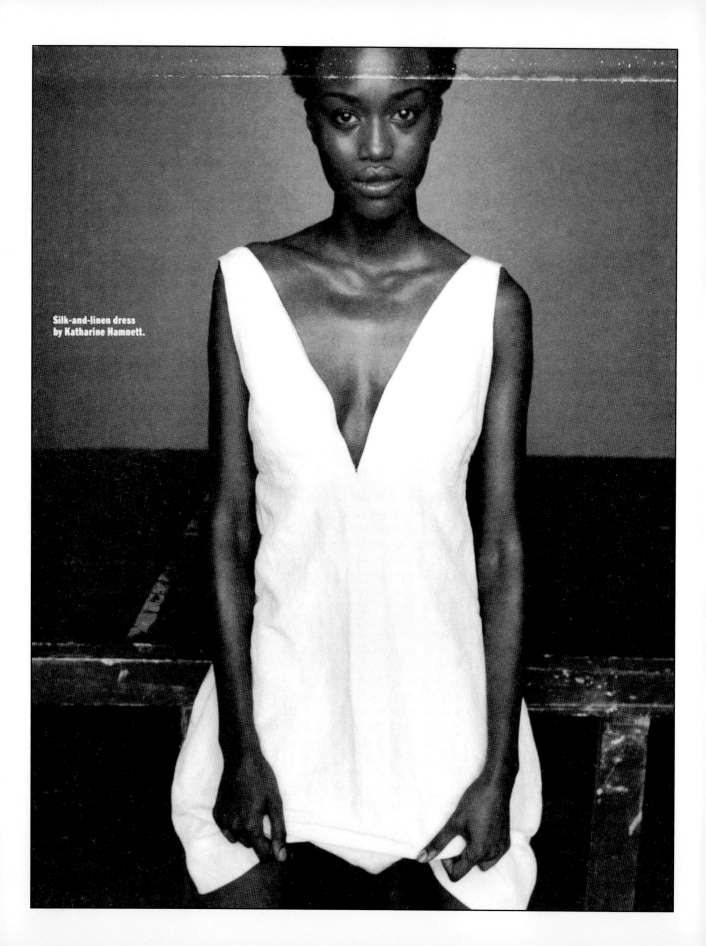

Silk-and-linen dress
by Katharine Hamnett.

A Personal Tribute to
Lois Samuels
Persona Extraodinaire

By Kingsley Cooper

I first met Lois at the Hampton High School for Girls in the St. Elizabeth countryside in Jamaica, while a fourteen year old schoolgirl there. Even then, her unusual beauty, sparkling personality and innate sense of style stood out. We met during Pulse's first ever **Model Search** and Lois' innocence, despite all the flair, was as obvious as it was charming and captivating.

Lois has gone on to become one of the supermodels, immediately recognizable throughout the international fashion world. In a fickle, unpredictable business, she has succeeded as much for her beauty and talent as she has for her abiding faith and powerful connection with the positive spiritual forces of the universe.

Undaunted by setbacks and motivated by rejection, her dedication and commitment to success are shining qualities that make her an outstanding example of the new woman of the world, of the Caribbean and of her native Jamaica where she is an inspiration to many and a role model to countless more.

Lois is also unique because her talent knows no bounds — model, charmer, artiste, writer, poet, painter, designer... Her little girl naivety, wisdom beyond her years, honesty and directness all add up to a peaceful, happy optimist, a result even more remarkable given the many apparent paradoxes that are a part of her being.

Having shared many of Lois' struggles, it has been my pleasure to rejoice in her successes. I look forward to the many dimensions of her success which I know will unfold in the years to come as she lives her multi-faceted life in what is, has been, and will continue to be a fascinating and brilliant career.

With the publication of this book, her real life drama continues to unfold. It is but another triumph along the road which I am sure will be a long and exciting journey to serendipity.

Lois is the very epitome of the great Romantic ideal in an age of cynicism. She has the daring never to compromise those ideals. This embodiment borne out in her philosophy of life is most aptly described in the words of Romantic poet, John Keats:

> 'Beauty' is truth, truth beauty,' — that is all
> Ye know on earth, and all ye need to know.

KINGSLEY COOPER
Kingsley Cooper is head of the **Pulse Model Agency** *which discovered Lois in Jamaica. He is also Executive Chairman of the Jamaica based* **Pulse Entertainment Group**.

Contents

as a flower blossoms
anchored in good soil
and nurtured in love
it becomes
it uncoils
and the beauty evolves

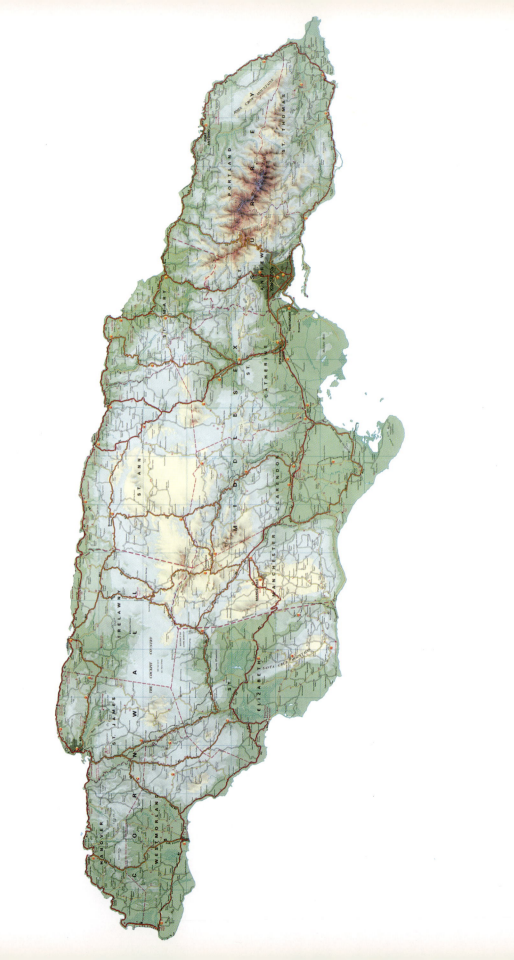

The Way It Was

As a young Jamaican girl, I grew up in the rural parish of St. Elizabeth located in the southern part of the island. My family was a small one consisting of my only sister Judine, my parents and myself. I will say my only sister Judine, for that is all I want to believe, even though I know my dear father has been busy over the years creating more "copies" of himself.

I was what you would call the 'black sheep' of my family. As long as I can remember my interests and needs were totally different to theirs and the other people I encountered daily. I simply found their way of living too predictable. For years their weekday routine remained unchanged; from waking up to the distant crowing of the cock each morning to listening to Alan Magnus in the Morning on Radio Jamaica and Rediffusion (RJR), with advertising jingles I had heard since I was three; to travelling the same long and tiny pot-holed route to work each morning, competing with Mr. Henry's market bus, for some space on the road, all the while conversing with the same people from the same work place. This was totally mundane to me.

This dull routine was broken by some variation during the weekends. Saturdays saw women who could afford it, going to one of the three hair salons. They would stand around in the sparsely seated parlour, gossiping and watching people go by while they waited to be the next victim of Miss Scuff, the hairdresser, as she scurried to process the strands on their beautiful heads, while unashamedly crucifying their scalps in order for them to look 'more presentable' . . . or 'less black' (as I would say) . . . When all is done, they would finally leave, looking almost the same as when they walked in.

In Santa Cruz, the capital, one could rarely find magazines showing positive images of dark-skinned women that would enhance the belief that society would accept and appreciate them the way they were. Not even the one television station I grew up watching showed beautiful or natural positive images of black people. So, young as I was, I could almost understand their crisis and their incessant desire to change their physical appearance.

Sunday mornings would see the same ladies, up early, grating coconuts for the usual rice and peas with chicken dinner, before going to the same Baptist church, to hear a sermon comprising of the same words as the one four Sundays ago. As I grew up I became aware of these Baptist churches all over the island and realized the very important role they played in the abolition of slavery. Maybe even to this day we still listen to the same sermons the slaves first heard from those missionaries.

I still remember the Sunday sermons when the minister would display much rage towards the congregation as he sought their response to his threats of how lethal God could be and how damned their souls would be if they did not make it up to the altar. It was almost scary. I, in contrast, wondered how many souls I could help to save in a modest way, by forgetting the fire and brimstone sermons. For to me, my God was a good, compassionate and understanding God.

No matter how I tried to make an effort to see it as it was, everything seemed to me to be a recurring decimal, an endless process of unrelieved boredom. I thought that perhaps with age, I would grow to appreciate this way of living as it represented what is considered safe and stable, where in most cases, the 'lifestyle' is set by the family, the job, the social norms and neighbourly discourses.

I found that the idea of being free and taking chances always gave me an incredible surge of energy, but very little chance to expend it. The idea of travel and my continued choice of preferred isolation created for me a close relationship with God, and soon I found the idea of being a missionary and having to travel the world most appealing. I used to spend many days fantasizing about travelling into various communities and setting up tents in the grass lands to have devotions, and to really make a difference by drawing people to know a loving God, One that would eliminate pride or the fear of feeling threatened by omnipresent powers.

Living in the country in my early years I grew to love farming. I even went on to study Agricultural Science at Hampton, which I passed at the Caribbean Certificate Examination (CXC) level. I loved the smell of the earth and of cut grass. For me nothing beats the smell of my Jamaican dirt after the rain has blessed the freshly cut grass and left it to bask in the sun's haze. (I guess it is a bit of the farm girl in me, which makes me love those things, all from growing up intermittently on my Dad's farm.) There is also my inherent affinity with Jamaica's flora and fauna. In all my travels, no dirt has ever had the depth of its fragrance, and no wind has ever caressed my skin and exhilarated my body like the Jamaican zephyr which would make the tall Jamaican grass sway and dance in its mellow way. This was most apparent in December, when the Christmas breeze would blow through St. Pauls where Dad's farm was or Top Hill, where my mother grew up. Neither New York's Central Park, nor London's Hyde Park nor Paris' le Jardin de Louvre, has ever given me that deja vu feeling which nature gives in Jamaica.

Many times in those days I would wonder, if I became a farmer, would my crops flourish, would my cattle be frail four legged creatures or not. Would they be longing for freedom from our waiting stomachs as I yearned for freedom from the monotonous life that stood before me? I guess it was probably no different for the animal as it was for me. Indeed, interestingly, there was no rebellion within me, just a quiet confidence, waiting for the road ahead to take its shape and form.

I wondered if I became an artist, would the world accept my concept and expression of life? Would I be able to survive?

I had a problem with what the people around me considered art. If they did not see the picture of a man with his dog, or a table with fruits, and a basket of flowers, in the brightest reds, yellows and greens, it was not art. Art was only what they could relate to from what they saw on an everyday basis. Art was not what you could feel, like it was for me.

These were some of the thoughts, very private thoughts which I shared exclusively with my God and my daily journals, in which I kept records of my thoughts and prayers. This is something that I still do today and often re-read to reflect on the various periods of my life and to draw my own inspiration.

During those early days, I designed clothes while secretly hoping to one day be a fashion designer. I remember one Sunday evening, when I was about eighteen, my sister's co-worker Joyce, asked me for a design. I was so thrilled knowing that someone had an interest in what I was doing that I dashed off for my sketch pad and quickly pulled out a beautiful long slinky black dress, with white bands around the top of it, to show her. She left with her sketch. I still do not know if she used my design at all, but . . .

Black and white were my colours at the time, not like today where I tend to wear only dark or muted shades. I believe I cannot think in colours even though I know dark-skinned people look beautiful it bright colours. I, on the contrary, almost feel like a fish out of water when wearing them. So at that time anything I sketched was black or black and white.

Was I telling myself then, that this was going to be my world?

Eventually, I had this same dress made by a local seamstress, Winnie, and wore it myself in the Jamaica Fashion Model Pageant. I believed it looked incredible and when I hit the runway for the show, it was confirmed, as I was greeted by a resounding applause from the audience.

In addition to designing, I filled in my boring spare time writing poetry, which I recited over the phone to the baby brother of my sister's classmate, Riggley (who I had a hard time convincing that I really wrote them). As an almost natural extension of my creativity, I started playing music, and ended up mastering the keys of a few musical instruments. I especially liked the piano and the recorder. I occasionally performed piano pieces at school devotions at Hampton, which was a continuity of my performance at Santa Cruz Preparatory when at the tender age of eleven still tall and skinny I played for my school graduation. I still remember how proud my father was. It was also at this school that I had my first taste of ballet,

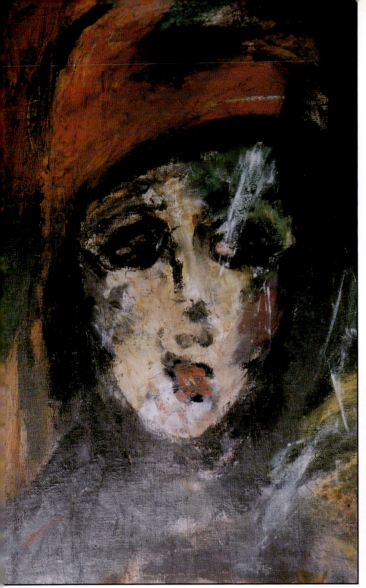

pretending we/don't exist/makes seeing us/
from the outside/desirable.

tears/only help/seeds of sorrow to grow

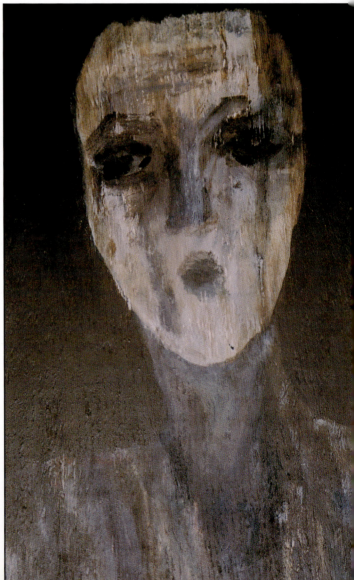

which was even further down the end of the totem pole, as it was considered a real dead end being considered a profession or pursuit not worth contemplating. Anyway, I would eagerly wait for Sunday evenings to put on my mother's panty hose stockings, tune the radio station to Sunday Evening Classics on the usual RJR, and run around on the barbecue (which was really the concrete surface for drying coffee and pimento), dancing, for the occasional eyes of my mother and sister.

With my poetry, my painting, my music and designing, I became the proverbial armchair traveller. For in a tiny country like Jamaica the chances of ever becoming a professional ballet dancer, poet or painter were restricted. And indeed the creative world was one not to be ventured into. Such pursuits were not to be encouraged by most families. The usual course to be followed for a young Jamaican woman after finishing her schooling was to find a job, get married and start having children.

Taking to the stage and to a creative career, even in music or dance or drama was totally unheard of, much less the one I eventually chose. But things slowly started to change over the years, especially since Bob Marley helped to put the face of Jamaica on the map through music. In the world of fashion there was the success of Grace Jones, model turned actress and eventually singer, and Pulse model, Kimberly Mais who had a lucrative career in Japan. And the continued fight by Pulse Investment Ltd./Model Agency (the one that discovered me), to establish the world of fashion as a business in Jamaica, has been considerably successful in gaining public acceptance for the beauty industry. To be a model is no longer considered a dead end street. This is quite a milestone for the beauty industry.

to be here
and not be apart of it all
is freedom
to have everything
and possess nothing
is the greatest freedom

y approach to life and its creative challenges was not clearly understood by my family and caused a lot of tension. With my mother, there were many confrontations. She was what I would call a 'Cedar tree of Lebanon', tall, very strong, yet very gentle and loving. She was a teacher for over three decades in a government school and was a calm yet strict disciplinarian, a trait I figured she brought home from having to deal with so many unruly children in the terribly overcrowded Jamaican classrooms. For her, seeing her daughter heading into a sea of unpredictables was not something easy to bear. She knew the importance of having a good education to go into the world with, and maybe from seeing the successes of children she had taught over her many years made her desire the same for me along the same traditional and unending path.

My father, a farmer was the one mostly responsible for my venture in the field of modelling. He had a better understanding of me. On the other hand, he always appeared in many ways to want the opposite of what my mother would desire. Apart from our love of farming, taking care of the red and black pole cows and various fruit trees on the property, my Dad and I shared many similar interests. We liked certain foods like our national Jamaican dishes, ackee and saltfish with sweet steamed bammies, sugar cane and curried lobster to name a few. We loved antique things: cars and houses, like the one we lived in, which was built in 1863 by the English settlers who I still believe live there along with the souls of the tortured slaves. I remember having encountered a few of them roaming in and out of the house when I was growing up. There was a particular one who would sit at one of the doors leading to the bathroom from the room my sister and I shared. I would be so scared that even the dim glow of the kerosene lamp my Mom would leave in the bathroom, would not give me enough guts to go for a pee. I would have to wake my sister up and beg her to follow me five steps to the bathroom which she rarely did. She was not afraid of what she could not see, and still isn't.

Jamaica is renowned for many old estate houses owned by distinguished families. The Barrett's of Whimpole Street after whom Barrett Town in Montego was named is one such family. Dad and I shared other interests apart from old houses. We also loved music, whether it be classicals (of Tchiakovsky or Schubert) or the strong chanting rhythm of Burning Spear. My Dad followed up on my musical interest and bought me a second-hand piano on my eleventh birthday. I remember how excited I was about it; I could not wait to get around it and play. The odds of having a piano at home in Jamaica at that time was one in ten thousand. On special, but too few Sundays he would listen to me play; it was a rare event, as we shared two different roofs. He would spend most of his time on the farm in St. Pauls, Manchester, while my sister and I lived with my mother in the warm valley of Santa Cruz. My family had what I would call a 'distant closeness'. To us, the phrase 'ever so near' could not apply and indeed 'distance did not affect the

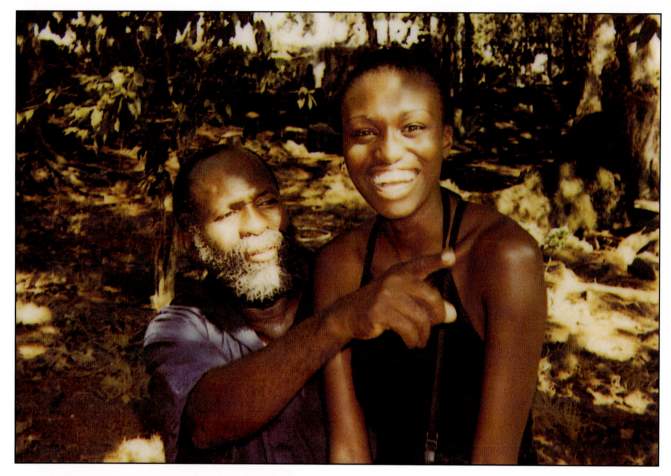

posing on the farm with Daddy in St. Pauls, Manchester.

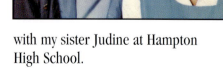

with my sister Judine at Hampton High School.

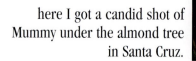

here I got a candid shot of Mummy under the almond tree in Santa Cruz.

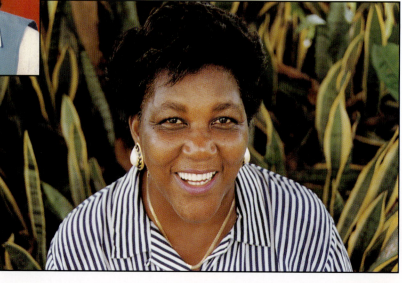

understanding we had'. But even though there was this geographical separation, whenever the opportunity was found, it was to me, my Dad gave a lot of support.

In retrospect, though my mother was initially in disagreement with my choice of career, today I see it as an element that only helped to make me into a stronger person.

My older sister, by a year, Judine was neither for nor against anything, but she supported me in her own subtle way, and still does. I guess she just left me to follow my own path, and I left her to follow hers.

I still vividly recall the beautiful sunlit morning in 1988, when all but fourteen and a student at the Hampton High School in Malvern, (one of the most respected girls' high schools in the island), I came charging from that edifice called Valhalla, which was used as the piano room, and where I studied music alone with Mr. Mullings my teacher.

Valhalla! How strange a name this is in the Jamaican countryside. History has it that Valhalla was built by an old Englishman, who settled in Jamaica and patterned the culture of Hampton School to that of an old English school. The school had in the past only tutored children of British descent, or white children, but in 1962 when Jamaica attained its independence, that, like many other things, changed. But not the fable of the old Englishman of Hampton who, it was said, had buried his five wives under each of the five rooms at Valhalla, as he loved music (they unlike me will never be free!...).

So it was on that day, in my flight to reality, I was spotted by Kingsley Cooper of Pulse Model Management as he scouted for contestants for the Jamaica Fashion Model Pageant. I had heard and read in advertisements about Pulse: it was the only established agency in the island and had in time become affiliated with international fashion agencies. In expanding the agency's outreach, Mr. Cooper had moved from only settling for girls in Kingston and the surrounding areas, and reached out to the country areas. This was a marketing thrust to garner new talent from across the island. Oblivious to all this, and focusing on a normal day, I almost certainly did not expect to be chosen by Pulse on that blessed morning.

Being naturally tall and slender I was always being told to consider modelling, but I never thought of myself as beautiful: to be truthful, I was a bit shy and very insecure about my looks. On reflection the society I grew up in, dictated it that way. And it never ceases to amaze me how mentally enslaved we still can be by believing one is less beautiful and less important due to the pigmentation of the skin. The approach of many Jamaicans towards one's colour still seems a topic to be buried but happily there are signs that we understand the presence of it more now, even though the issue will not be resolved in a short time. As our Bob Marley said, "Emancipate yourselves from mental slavery; none but ourselves can free our minds . . ."

Needless to say I was more than elated when Pulse, from the entire school of hundreds, selected only two girls, one of whom happened to be me and the other, Nikki Swaby.

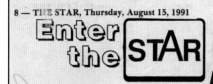

Enter the STAR COMPETITION
AND PICK THE WINNER OF THE

JAMAICA F
PAGE

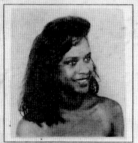

NICOLE BAILEY – 5' 8" 14 YRS.
RED ROSE TEA

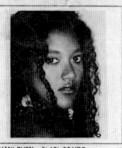

SHANI CHEN – 5' 10" 20 YRS.
AMMAR'S

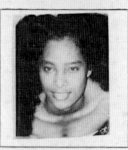

WENDY DALEY – 5' 7" 16 YRS.
SAMURAI INVESTMENTS

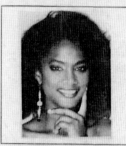

LAURIE ANN DOUGLAS – 5' 7" 15 YRS.
HEDONISM II

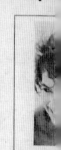

KAREN DUHA
VAZ ENT

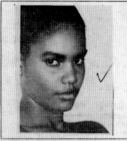

KAREN BROWN – 5' 8" 20 YRS.
SPECS

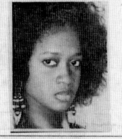

LAUREL BROWN – 5' 9½" 25 YRS.
DANWILL'S MOTOR & SERVICE

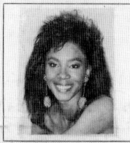

STRYCEN DUSSARD – 5' 10½" 19YRS.
GARFIELD'S DIVING STATION

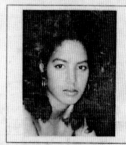

SIMONE FORBES – 5' 7" 17 YRS.
CREATIVE KITCHENS

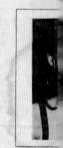

ROMAE GORD
CREMO L

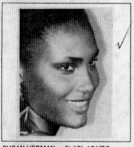

SUSAN HERMAN – 5' 10" 17 YRS.
PETCOM

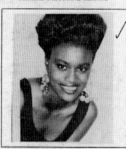

LOIS SAMUELS – 5' 10½" 18 YRS.
TIMES STORE

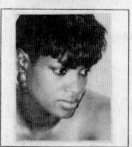

ZONYA RODNEY – 5' 8" 24 YRS.
LANDER

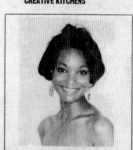

JACKIE PALMER – 5' 10" 22 YRS.
HARMONY INVESTMENTS

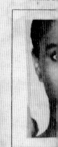

JUDY SUTHER
MICHAEL

DON'T MISS

GRAND FINALS

SAT. 24th AUG.

PULSE, 38 Trafalgar Road.

Special Feature

Highlights from the

MALE FASHION REVUE

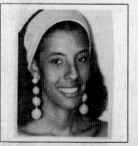

JANILLE HOLUNG – 5' 7" 22 YRS.
KEY INSURANCE

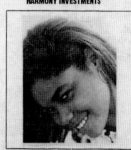

RACQUEL HUTCHINSON – 5' 10" 18 YRS.
PLEASURE TOURS

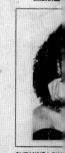

SUZANNE LOW
SARAH OF

BETTER THAN EVER !

finalists for the 1991 Jamaica fashion model Pageant.

HION MODEL
T 1991

AND WIN

- **FIRST PRIZE**
  $1,000 CASH
  FROM **PULSE**

- **SECOND PRIZE**
  1 CASE OF
  Mountain Peak
  INSTANT COFFEE
  EXTRAORDINARY

- **THIRD PRIZE**
  1 CASE OF
  SMIRNOFF
  GOOD FRIENDS AND SMIRNOFF
  – BEYOND THE ORDINARY

- **FOURTH PRIZE**
  6 MONTHS SUPPLY OF
  Soflan
  THE GENTLE DETERGENT

- **FIFTH PRIZE**
  GIFT PACKAGE OF
  OPTIMUM
  Condition by Soft Sheen

- **SIXTH PRIZE**
  6 MONTHS SUPPLY OF
  SEA BREEZE

PLUS CASES OF **ting** & GIFT PACKAGES OF **OZ** & **Posner**

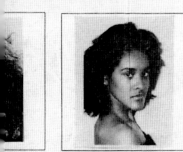

YRS.
JANICE DUNKLEY – 5' 8" 16 YRS.
HILLCREST VILLAGE

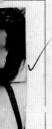

8 YRS.

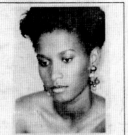

BRIDGETTE McDONALD – 5' 7" 20YRS.
CARIBBEAN LIFESTYLES

CLAIRE ANN O'MEALLY – 5' 10" 20YRS.
AMBI

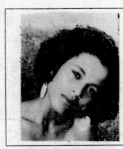

KELLY SCOTT – 5' 10" 22 YRS.
TANG

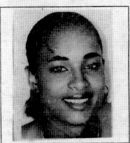

NARINE GRINDLEY – 5' 7" 16 YRS.
HUNGRY JACK

20 YRS.
VICE CENTER

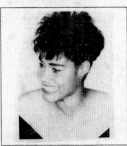

DONALDENE WAUGH – 5' 9" 22 YRS.
LA ROOSE

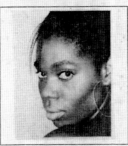

SONIA WALKER – 6' 21 YRS.
COUPLES

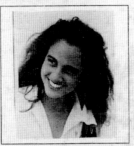

DIANNE THOMPSON – 5' 7" 16 YRS.
EXCLUSIVE GARDENS

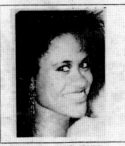

ARLENE ROSE – 5' 8½" 19 YRS.
ACROPOLIS DISCO

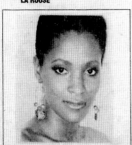

7 YRS.
SANDRA MAXWELL – 5' 7½" 25 YRS.
GUARDIAN INS. BROKERS

PHOTOS:
Michelle Jackson

MAKE-UP
Annette Meeks

RULES

1. PHOTOGRAPHS OF THE FINALISTS WILL APPEAR IN THE STAR & THE SUN. MAGAZINE 3 TIMES WEEKLY.
   YOU ARE ASKED TO JUDGE WHICH OF THE FINALISTS WILL WIN THE JAMAICA FASHION MODEL PAGEANT 1991.

2. FILL OUT THE ENTRY COUPON INDICATING YOUR CHOICE, YOUR OWN NAME AND ADDRESS, AND MAIL TO:
   "THE STAR PICK THE WINNER COMPETITION" THE GLEANER COMPANY LIMITED, 7 NORTH STREET, KINGSTON OR DROP IN SPECIAL BOXES PROVIDED AT THE COMPANY'S OFFICES IN KINGSTON, 7 NORTH STREET AND IN MONTEGO BAY, 34 UNION STREET.

3. FINAL DATE FOR RECEIPT OF ENTRIES IS SATURDAY AUGUST 23th 4:00 P.M.

4. EACH ENTRY MUST BE ON AN ORIGINAL STAR ENTRY COUPON.

5. THE FIRST PRIZE OF THE COMPETITION WILL GO TO THE FIRST CORRECT ENTRY OPENED, SECOND AND THIRD PRIZES WILL GO TO THE NEXT TWO CORRECT ENTRIES OPENED.

6. THE COMPETITION IS OPEN TO THE PUBLIC WITH THE EXCEPTION OF THE EMPLOYEES OF THE GLEANER COMPANY LIMITED, IT'S ADVERTISING AGENCY OR PULSE LIMITED.

FILL IN THIS COUPON

Pick the Winner of the
Jamaica Fashion Model Pageant 1991

NAME:..

ADDRESS:..

THE JUDGES WILL CHOOSE...........................

I remember how it was such a big deal for the entire school population. It was so much "the talk," that it opened my eyes to the fact that almost every girl seemed to have the dream of wanting to be a model or a beauty queen. Funny enough, despite all my creative appreciation towards the arts and music, I cannot remember fantasizing about being a model. I did a few fashion shows in my community, and at the schools' fair. Even though I never considered myself beautiful, I always responded on the basis of my height and physique.

Once I was offered the opportunity from Pulse, I was curious to see how far it could take me. And so as a logical extension, I became a part of the Pulse family and entered the 1988 Annual Jamaica Fashion Model Pageant.

It was an awkward yet exciting feeling during those first few days when I was exposed to the nuances and whims of Jamaica's modelling world. Barry Moncrieffe was the designer whom I represented, on my first appearance for Pulse in August 1988. I wore a beautiful little white linen dress, I remember.

I recall how my mother, who I must give some credit for sticking it out, took me by taxi a few times on that two-hour trip from Santa Cruz into Kingston, as she was advised by my Dad not to drive in the city. Dad felt it was too dangerous for us both to drive in the city, (people from the country always saw the big city as being unsafe) but the other reason, which was, the real reason I believe, was that my mother's Audi car could barely take her to and from Mandeville, which was only about twenty five miles from Santa Cruz, without the radiator screaming, let alone Kingston, which was a hundred miles away. On the actual weekend, when the show was held, my family was there for the event. Nothing is better than having the presence of the entire family, as I now know, since I do not enjoy that experience any more and miss their complete presence.

Mother had remained unchanged and unenthusiastic about me being a part of this "masquerade," as she would call it. And even though I was not placed in this my first attempt, it made no difference to us as a family unit but gave me the most interesting experience of my up to then, predictable life.

It was my first time being in a 'pool' filled with so much ego. The competitive air was so strong that I felt dizzy—dizzy from insecurity. Perhaps this was because I had not yet learned to totally love and appreciate myself. First of all, I was very dark-skinned and all around me and in the big city being light-skinned with softer textured hair was obviously the "in" thing. Secondly, I was a 'country girl' coming to the city; and thirdly neither my parents nor I were rich. It was the first time I realized, how lost and shallow people can become, placing emphasis on that which is purely physical.

For the first time I saw 'vanity' the 'disease'.

Out of that experience, and my first exposure to this new world of fashion, my attention to school and school work was affected and my grades dropped drastically. In a few short months I saw myself fall from

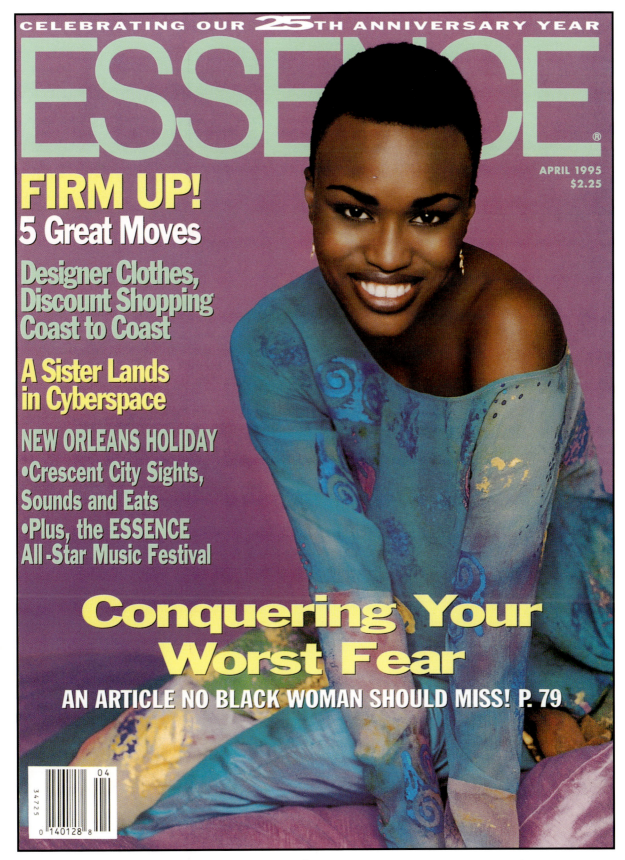

the cover of *Essence,* 1995.

being in the top ten of my class to being placed twenty-third or twenty-second. I remember how terribly shocked I was. I guess I was flying in that sky of fantasies, so I immediately dived down and continued to battle to improve my school grades. Putting the temporary modelling world behind me, I achieved seven subjects, including two distinctions at O levels, before going on to Knox Community College in Clarendon, to do my A levels.

But the years for my girlhood desire to challenge the unknown returned and I barely did a year of studying at Knox when that urge to be a free spirit overcame the torture and boredom of trying to accomplish tasks that were set for me to follow. I also was not enjoying the place called Knox College, for the people constantly mocked me about my physique. At that time there was a musician known only as 'Red Dragon', who came out with a disrespectful tune called 'Cu..cumm, cumm', which portrayed a negative and comical image of slender women, or what he called 'meagre women'. It stressed the fact that when these women moved, their bones rattled making terrible noises.

I really took this teasing and the song so seriously, that there were days I would come home on the verge of tears. Daily, I publicly "fried" myself in the midday sun by wearing oversized jackets to cover my embarrassment.

On my own initiative, four years later in 1991, having just spent a little over a year at Knox, I re-entered the Jamaica Fashion Model Pageant at eighteen. I figured that if this was the medium through which I could get out to see the world and enjoy new experiences this was It. My mind was crystal clear and my singular purpose was success. Even though my decision was not encouraged by anyone and I was alone with my decision, I was determined to make something of it, this time. I prayed constantly for a medium to get out, and I believed God was directing me through this path.

I was an instant crowd favourite this time around. I experienced goose pimples as thunderous applause greeted me each time I hit the ramp in clothes made by Arlene Richards, who like Barry Moncrieffe, my first designer, was a dancer and costume designer for the National Dance Theatre Company (NDTC), Jamaica's internationally acclaimed dance company. What I modelled was a golden Egyptian-styled dress with a beaded head cap, which I still keep in the last drawer in my bedroom in Santa Cruz. It was beautiful. That night, I was placed in the top ten, in the eighth position, to be exact, and I was judged as being the most dynamic model. Romae Gordon was the lucky winner that year.

The structure of the competition, however, was designed not only to focus on the winner, but to give an opportunity to the others. So, a few months later, as is customary, a happy group of enthusiastic and anxious finalists from this competition, along with Kingsley Cooper made its annual trip to agencies in Europe and America.

I felt I was flying through the gates of freedom. This was similar to the freedom I encountered one

Sunday evening, after one of our dogs had aggravated a mother cow and her calf who reacted in typical calf-like behaviour. My sister, myself and the mongrel dog fled down the little hill for the sake of our feeble little lives scared as hell, but running for freedom which I found at the side of a tank. Having secured the eighth position now, intensified my intention to put my face on the map of 'black' models internationally. I guess each girl had her own thoughts that night, picturing her success, and hoping all would work positively for her.

But reality can be cruelly stark when you enter the world's market place.

Paris was our first stop. Here I was in Paris, the centre of fashion, which I was ready to take on like a tropical hurricane and only one agency showed a tinge of interest in me? Maybe it was my hair, maybe it was my smile or maybe I was really ugly after all . . . It was most depressing. And so we went on to London and the same thing happened. With only one agency showing a tiny bit of interest, nothing happened. What was going on? I guess they did not see what I believed I had to offer. So, off we went to New York. We stayed at the Hotel Edison, in the 'heart of the Big Apple'—Times Square. Perhaps being bruised by all my rejections I found nothing impressive. Not the bright lights, or the multitude of people. Not the abundance of stores, or those tall black 'drop dead' gorgeous guys who looked like basketball players; or the Rastafarians, the ones I was crazy about.

To think about it nothing impressed me throughout the entire trip: not walking down past the Louvre on Rue de Rivoli and hearing French, the language of love, nor seeing people eating at the smart outdoor cafes while smoking their gouloises in their expensive Chanel outfits and Dior shades. In London, maybe I thought the double-deckered buses were cute and the music groovy. But New York! . . . The only square in the world where every culture fused, and I was blind from concentration. I needed an agency to represent me so badly, I could not see what New York had to offer. The days went by, and saw me going in and out of agencies, the picture and the words becoming more and more predictable, "You have an interesting look, but . . ." Although Pulse was there for me as a Mother Agency, they were still feeling their own way into the world of fashion, trying to pass on their dreams and desires, no different than us, their models.

On my last day Tyronne Barrington and the owner of Bethann Management, Bethann Hardison, who then represented Roshumba and Tyson Beckford, decided to take an unexplained chance with me. I saw this as a miracle from God. Even though there was no contract signed, so eager was I that not having a contract did not matter to me. God had given the light and I was going to carry that torch. I knew no one in New York, did not have much money and really had no where to stay (since the agency did not at that time have accommodation for me in a model's apartment), but New York had to be the base, and it had to happen. I was not ready to go back to Jamaica. I was determined to make something of my presence in this world.

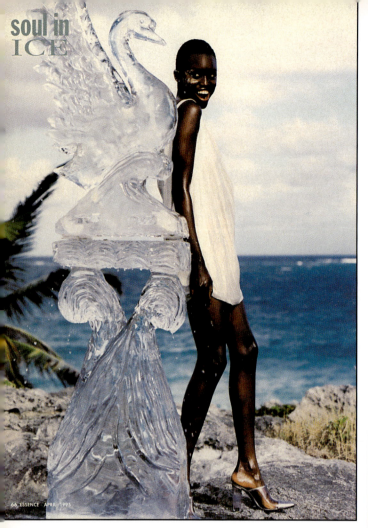

66. ESSENCE · APRIL 1995

Strong, clear hues beneath a blazing Barbados sun. For a touch of shine, nothing beats the luster of satin, the fabric of the season. Right: Lime-green satin jacket, $635, and A-line skirt, $168, Helen Storey. Photographed at Harry Smith Beach. Left: Silver satin tank dress, $220, Migoscha. Silver sandals, Sam & Libby. Cuff, Cara Croninger at Fragments. Photographed in Speightstown. ▷

some "Soul in Ice".
this was one of my favorite photo
shoots. we had an excellent crew.
Ruven Afanador was the photographer.

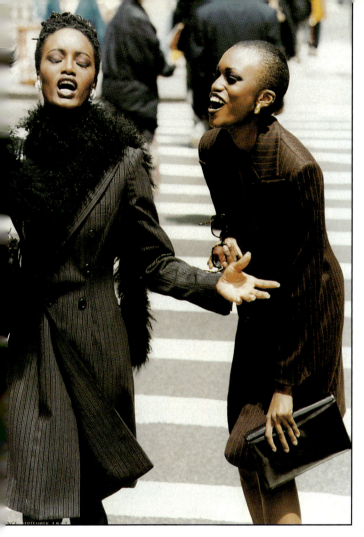

I again shot with *Essence* on location at Wall street with Haitian photographer, Marc Baptiste.

FLOURISHES THAT COUNT *The unexpected dash of a boa, a gutsy-colored top and the cool of an artsy cloche lend a striking edge to these suits. Far left: Double-breasted wool coat-dress, $1,695, Ralph Lauren Collection. Earrings, Lois Hill Accessories. Boa, Adrienne Landau. Handbag, Liz Claiborne. Hosiery, Essence. Left: Wool-and-Lycra striped jacket, $338, matching skirt, $118, and silk sweater, $175, Cynthia Rowley. Sunglasses, Oscar de la Renta. Earrings, Nikos at Edie Shane. Hosiery, Essence. Clutch, Judith Leiber. This page: Stretch suede jacket, $495, and skirt, $198, Cynthia Steffe. Burnout velvet shirt, $180, M.A.G. Hat, Carlos New York Hats. Boa, Adrienne Landau. Gloves, Carolina Amato. Handbag, Esprit. Hosiery, Hanes.* ▷

And so I started the long climb up the hill.

Though financially low, I remained in New York where my first interest came from the most popular magazine for the black woman, Essence. Their editors were testing a cover try with myself, and another Jamaican model who happened to be the winner of the first Supermodel of Jamaica Competition in 1990. As it turned out, I was not lucky to be on the cover then. But three years later, I achieved the cover status along with a beautiful story, Soul in Ice, for which we journeyed to my beautiful sister island, Barbados.

As was expected, there was very little money, and I had to find a way to stay on and pursue my dream and so I prayed for faith and found that indeed faith was the master. I located a friend of mine with whom I had attended Santa Cruz Prep School, Tanya Russell, and moved in with her and her Dad for a few long cold months. It was the first time, that I was experiencing winter. It was terrible; my so called winter leather jacket was a joke. The façade showed a leather jacket but inside I had sewn a sweater since there was no lining. I remember while making my rounds on castings, I would always be praying quite audibly, 'Father keep me warm, keep me warm, keep me warm . . .', and in turn to accompany my chant, I would make my wild imagination take me for a walk on Treasure Beach or through Santa Cruz market on a hot Saturday morning. Such positive reflections kept me going and always took me to my calls in one piece.

Tanya was a great friend to have, but I could not fight the sadness that would delve into my soul. I missed my family, and made endless collect calls sometimes twice per day to my mother. I received so much comfort from hearing her, and having her listen to me. Out of concern and her continued reservations about my career, she was beginning to encourage me to come back home and maybe go to school or something. She never said anything like " . . . I told you it wouldn't work or so..." But indirectly, I knew what she wanted, and she knew that I knew what she was trying to say. I missed the food, the boiled yams and dumplings with stewed beef. I missed the warmth of the people and the sun-boiled beauty of the St. Elizabeth plains. But then, at that time, I would rather continue in the cold of Fresh Meadows, Queens, than come home to Jamaica not accomplishing anything at all. Was this freedom after all?

before you
i am dust in the wind
i am nothing

.   .   .

*T*hose initial years from 1994-1995 were not easy. They were filled with much hardship. Financial instability made getting around the city and living in a comfortable environment quite difficult and at times nearly impossible. I was moving all over the city from the Robinsons' in Long Island, to the Russells' in Queens, to the Witters' in the Upper Bronx to the Samuels' in Upper Manhattan just to name a few, trying each time to be closer to the city. My place of rest was more than often in beds or sofas in the living rooms of people I barely knew, to cockroach infested rundown apartments as the one I stayed in on the Upper West Side of Manhattan. I never could stand roaches. Jamaican roaches, in fact, gave much more respect, compared to the New York roaches, who I have heard ever so often, 'cannot be beat'. In this apartment, I had to deal with these roaches as I had to deal with the sight of people running busily like ants once I stepped out the door. And no matter how many cans of Combat or Radar or sticky pad I bought, it made no difference to their ever increasing numbers. I became convinced that the roaches were family to the mother and daughter pair whom I was living with, as they were living quite comfortably with them prior to my arrival. I remember telling Marsha, "*. . . tell yu sister fi get out a mi tings . . .*" I rarely ate at home, if you could call this haven for cockroaches that. The competition was just too stiff, and my stomach too weak. A day's meal consisted of little, or sometimes nothing, yet, I was never ill. I suppose all the Jamaican callaloo and banana breakfasts did pay off after all.

I remained physically, emotionally and spiritually intact even under such terrible living conditions, never losing my touch with God. I would call on Him constantly and still at times record the blessings and happenings in my little books. I saw that the Great Force never leaves or forsakes you, nor allows you to handle more than you can possibly bear. I always believe that God only takes you to the limit to help make a better person out of you. And I believe also that sometimes God has His day, and the Devil has his way, as borne out in the life of Job.

I never mentioned any of my difficulties to my mother agency (Pulse), maybe it was my pride or maybe it was my faith for I saw that amidst it all, in cold winters there was always warmth. In sorrowful moments there was laughter. (I was always laughing anyway . . . I remember someone saying, "You can always know when Lois is coming . . . you see her teeth first," or I remember my mother once telling me that, 'I will end up like Brer Rabbit' if I did not stop the laughing). What can I say to that but declare I have a happy soul.

I always tried not to be too sad or worried for something would always be provided. With everything I could always see that silver glimmer of hope.

In recollection I value not having had great comfort in those days, because it makes me appreciate the smallest of things. It makes me appreciate a great meal at dinnertime, compared to a thin slice of pizza or an apple pie I had many times for dinner. It makes me see the importance of little things we take for granted, like having a long bath, talking to yourself and walking naked in your own space, having your independence and getting a good night's sleep. Simple things like that.

It is from being exposed to different experiences and events that you get a better understanding of yourself. You learn how to deal with rejections and how to be strong. I remember on one of my first castings, I went to see a photographer in New York's Chelsea district who had the nerve to tell me that I looked like a monkey. He even went on to describe the thickness of my lips, as he flipped through my portfolio. Instead of getting angry, yet, why get angry? I remember smiling in disbelief and at the same time feeling pity towards him. How can a rotten seed grow? I saw him two years later running around London, still trying to do the same thing, at the same level. He had not stepped up another rung on the ladder of life and was still not a recognised photographer.

This can be summed up in these four simple truths:

You learn about people.
Life is a circle.
What goes around, comes around.
Never render negative for negative. If you do, it makes you no better.

Much can be gained by learning to be intuitive, perceptive, appreciative and faithful. I guess that by the grace of God, I had the ability to attract and repel things. And l guess by the grace of God again, I was a dreamer, so I would be able to deal with certain situations after having confronted them before, even while in the deepest of sleep. I have seen the power in positive thinking, and l have seen the power one can have in controlling or predicting a situation, if you really focus on it and not rush into things.

Overall, there is just so much to see in the various cultures and beautiful souls of people and the ever-present miracles in life. Knowledge is infinite and if we have open minds to learn and absorb all there is for us to experience, our very lives are enriched.

Father You know the time
You know the space
there is not one thing unknown to You
You know my joy
You know my pain
You know it all

I recall my first job. It was the cover of a novel by April Sinclair Too Much Coffee Will Make You Black. It only showed my smile. I guess one should smile if coffee only makes one black. I suppose in St. Elizabeth, my parents must have had lots of coffee.

I was paid the princely sum of $150 but it was my first cover and I was very proud of it. I remember after I cashed that very first cheque, I went to a Mediterranean restaurant in Tribeca and ordered a 'cajun chicken breast' meal. I wanted to treat myself and experiment on other foods knowing the pleasure I get from eating.

During this period, I did a few test shots with photographers such as Tar and Kevin Weingart, (I have no idea where they are today). It was generally difficult for me to

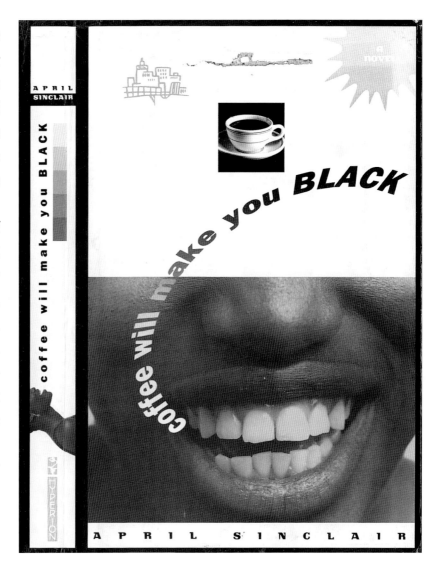

have a test done, since most photographers did not find me to be the type of material to do a test with. I was just not beautiful enough for them. Basically, I was very shy and so in most cases what I projected worked negatively against me. But the funny thing about it is, even though I was shy I was extremely confident; I really believed in myself, and I knew I could do it. So the daily rejections never curbed me into believing that I would ultimately fail.

The few tests I eventually did led to my first real photo shoot for Vibe magazine. The theme was a circus story, shot by Ruven Afanador using a real circus performer who took on the roles of a fire-eater, a tight rope-walker and a gymnast walking on stilts. My first photo shoot coupled with this being my first time seeing any act from a circus, right there on Pier 25 on the Hudson River in New York City, made me nervous, yet excited. It was indeed an exhilerating day, not to be forgotten.

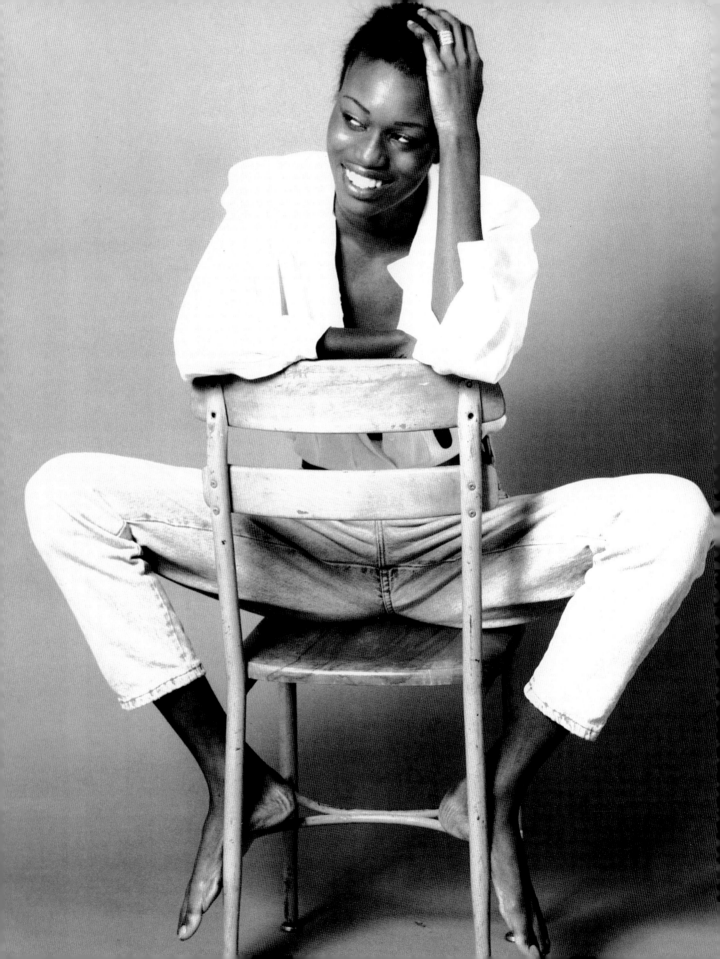

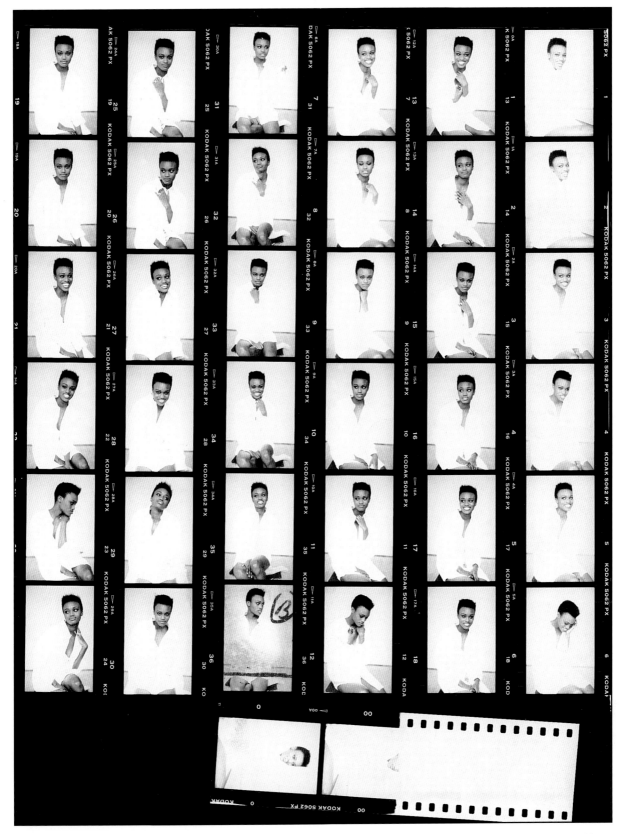

PHOTO: TAR.

PHOTO: Ken Weingart.

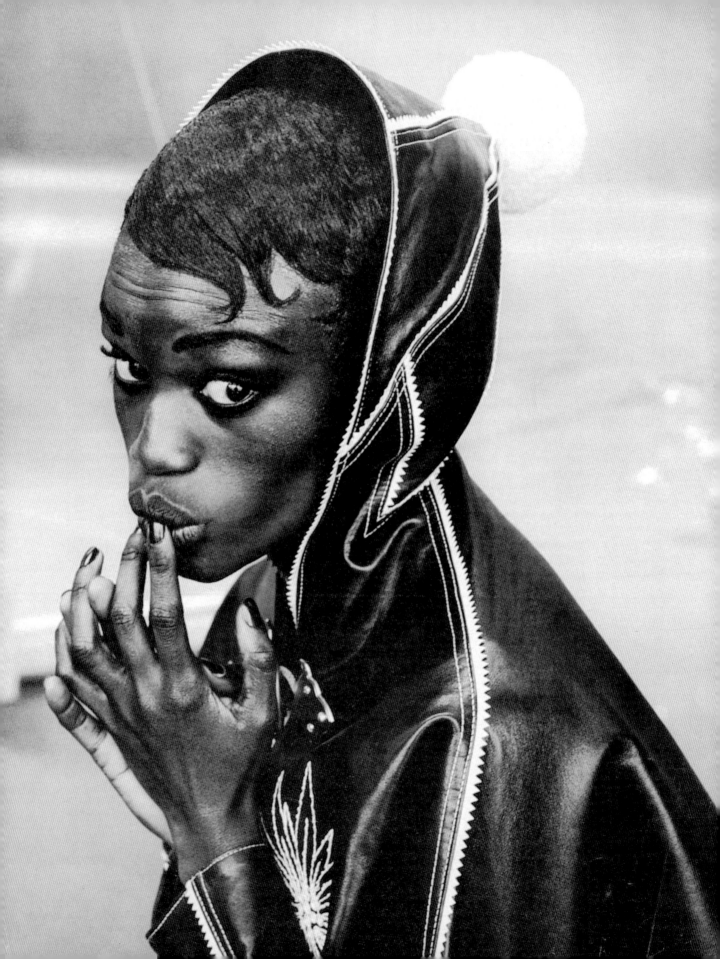

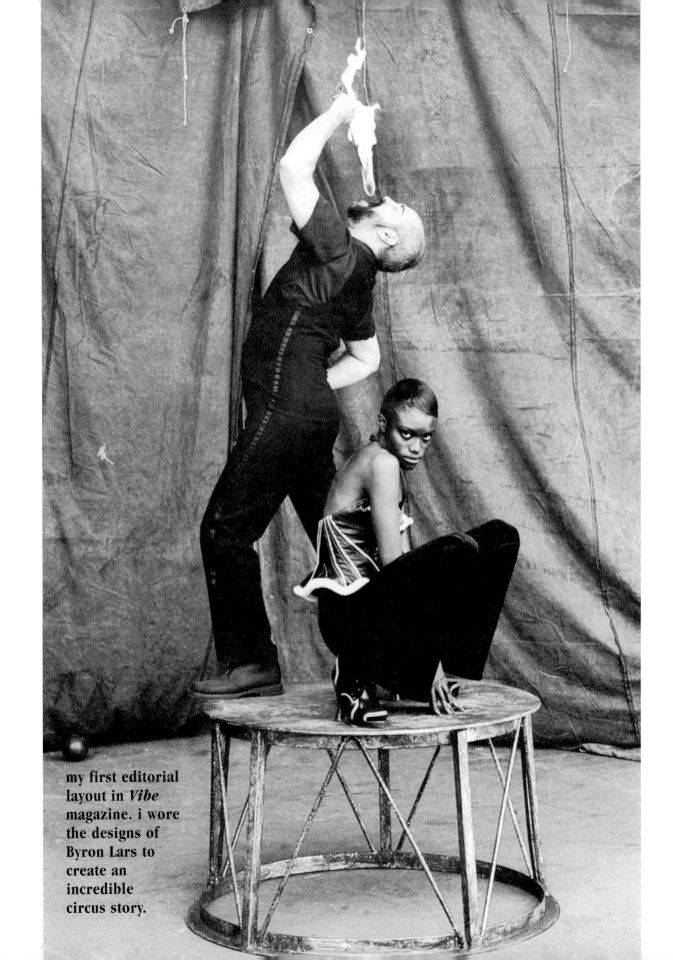

my first editorial layout in *Vibe* magazine. i wore the designs of Byron Lars to create an incredible circus story.

Compared to that splendid take off, the development of my career was slow. Needless to say, I was always without cash. I reluctantly returned home after realizing that things were not moving up in my mind or in my pocket. I ended up spending a few months, with my mother at home in Santa Cruz, until boredom overtook me and I set off to New York's hustle and bustle again. That was a mistake, for when I returned to the international market, it was like starting all over again. It is depressing and frustrating being in new country without family, without real friends and without healthy meals. Accentuating this situation is the inevitable freezing your derriere off in the cold weather. Thank God for His inspirations, I managed to write a lot of poems, poems that gave me comfort and inner strength, poems I would not have been able to write if I were living in a bed of roses.

When you find yourself in a situation like this, there is the innate urge to go home to your family, who will emotionally elevate you but in reality this damages your soul. Two alternatives present themselves. You either extinguish the fire within your soul or you charge it. I decided to charge it. I wanted to see the world, I wanted to feel the world and if I decided to do so through the life of a model, I had to fight and take the fire to great heights. I had to be in the eye of the storm to be a part of the storm. If I was not physically there where the action was, I would contribute to my own oblivion. The cliche, Out of sight - Out of mind, would then be inevitable. This was certainly not the picture I painted for myself.

I rolled up my sleeves, and got my act together. Soon I had a portfolio with a few editorials and was lucky to be booked for the Calvin Klien Campaign, CK One, shot by Steven Meisel. This drastically turned things around for me. Soon after, I was shooting with such photographers as Ellen von Unwerth, Jean Baptiste Mondino, Walter Chin, Albert Watson and working with renowned designers as Issey Miyake, Ralph Lauren, Christian Dior, Givenchy and Isaac Mizrahi. I hopped on and off planes and trains. I travelled to different parts of the world. I was happy that my dream was already beginning to come true. All that was left for me, after surmounting the hardships, was to learn what the real life of an international model demands.

Ckone, PHOTO: Steven Meisel.

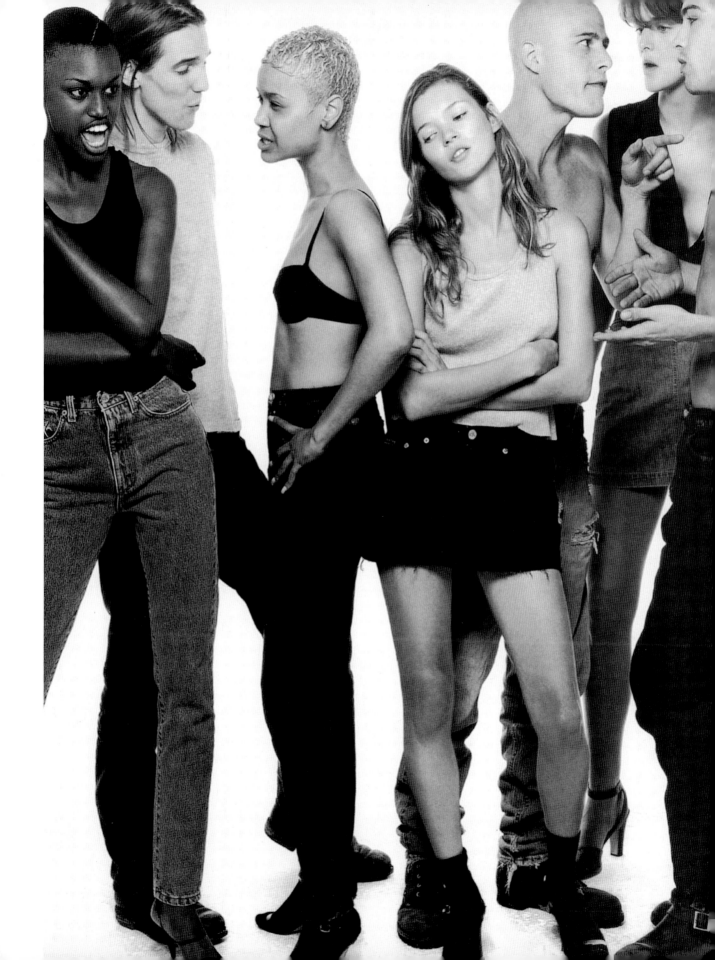

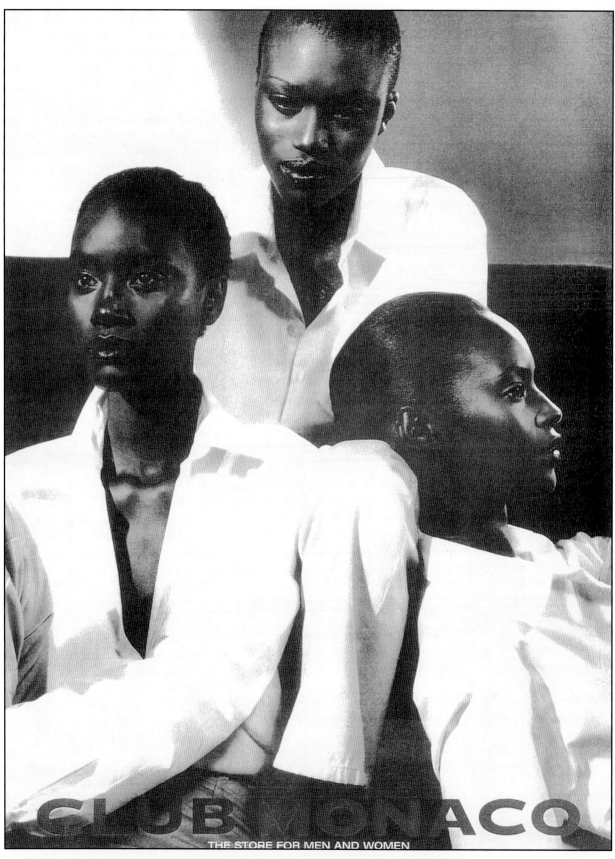

Club Monaco campaign, shot by Jamaica's own Walter Chin.

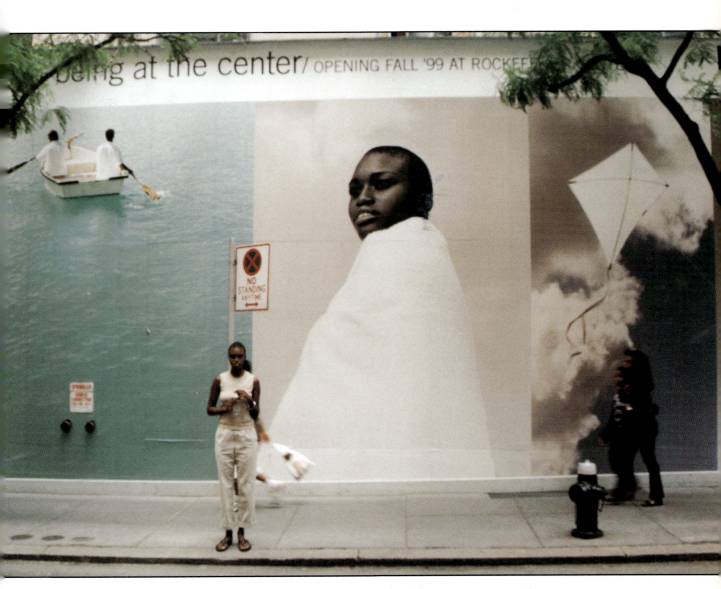

with Banana Republic billboard, at Rockerfeller Center, New York.

There are two new stars in the heavens...

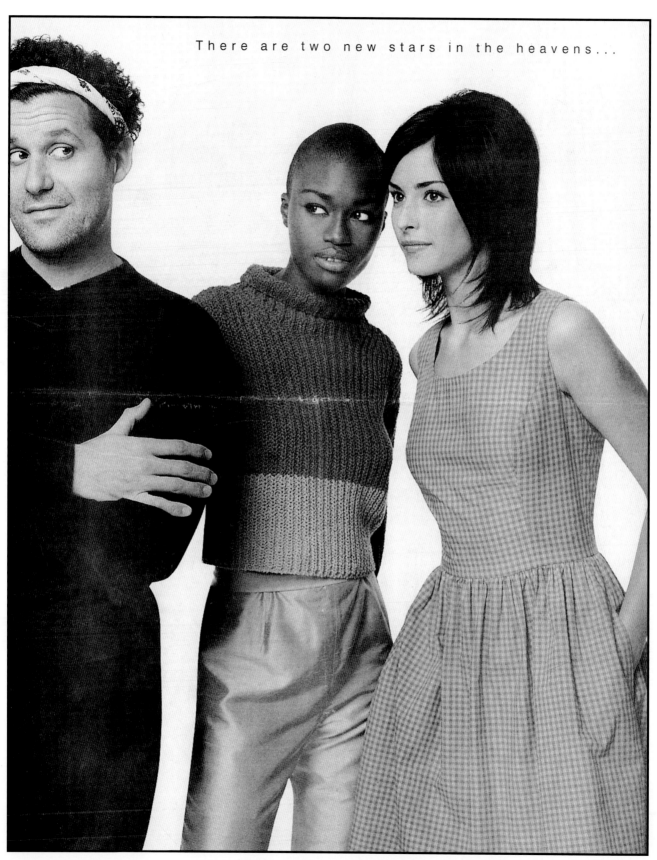

in New York Times with Isaac Mizrahi.

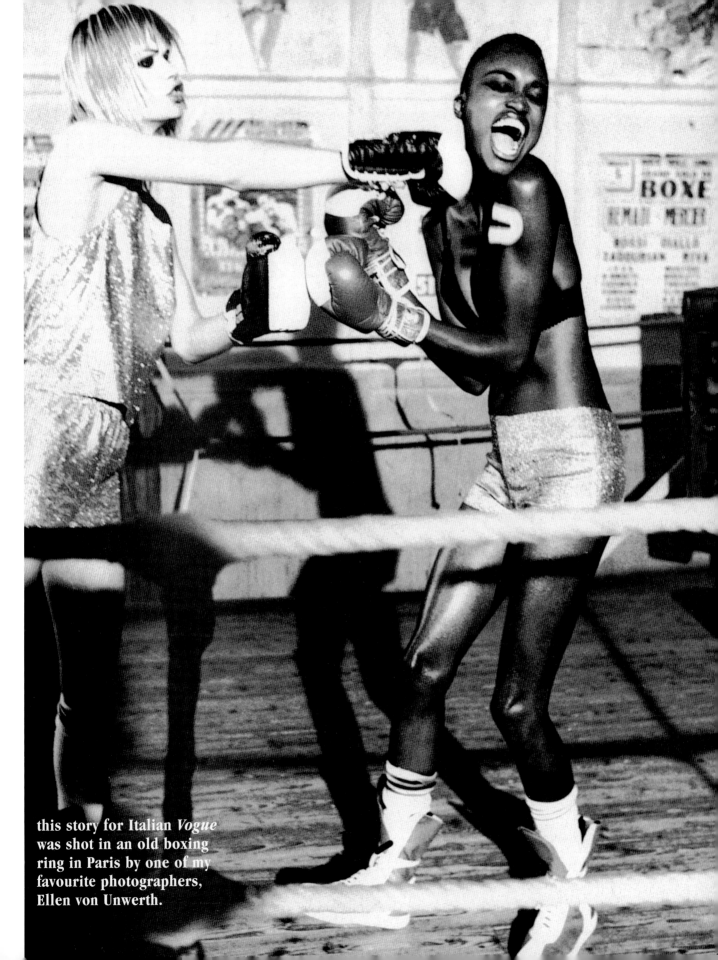

this story for Italian *Vogue* was shot in an old boxing ring in Paris by one of my favourite photographers, Ellen von Unwerth.

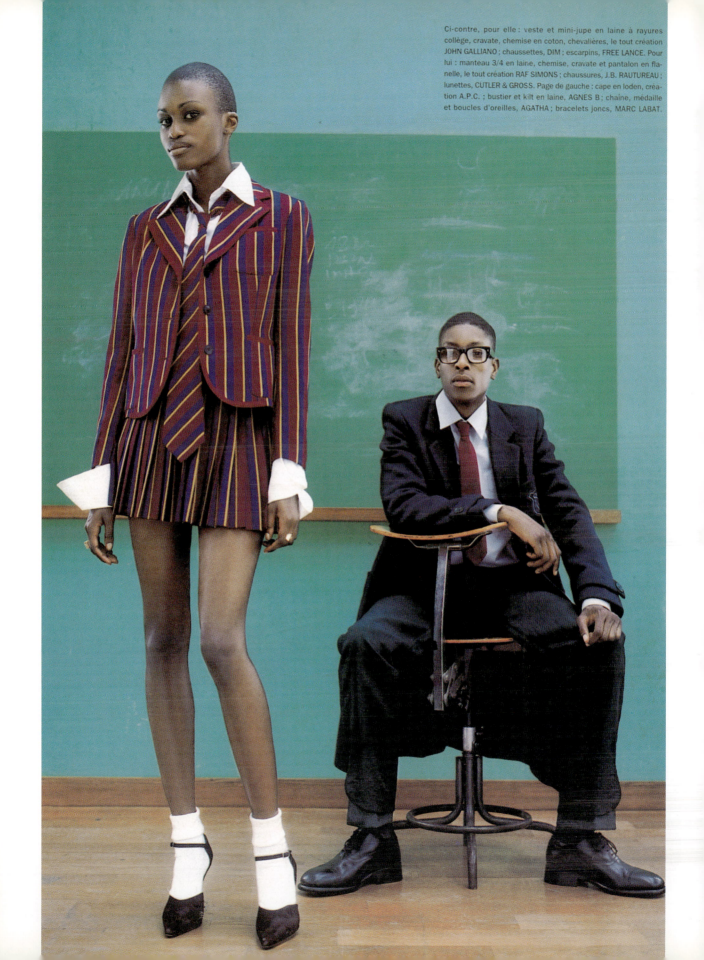

Ci-contre, pour elle : veste et mini-jupe en laine à rayures collège, cravate, chemise en coton, chevalières, le tout création JOHN GALLIANO ; chaussettes, DIM ; escarpins, FREE LANCE. Pour lui : manteau 3/4 en laine, chemise, cravate et pantalon en flanelle, le tout création RAF SIMONS ; chaussures, J.B. RAUTUREAU ; lunettes, CUTLER & GROSS. Page de gauche : cape en loden, création A.P.C. ; bustier et kilt en laine, AGNES B ; chaîne, médaille et boucles d'oreilles, AGATHA ; bracelets joncs, MARC LABAT.

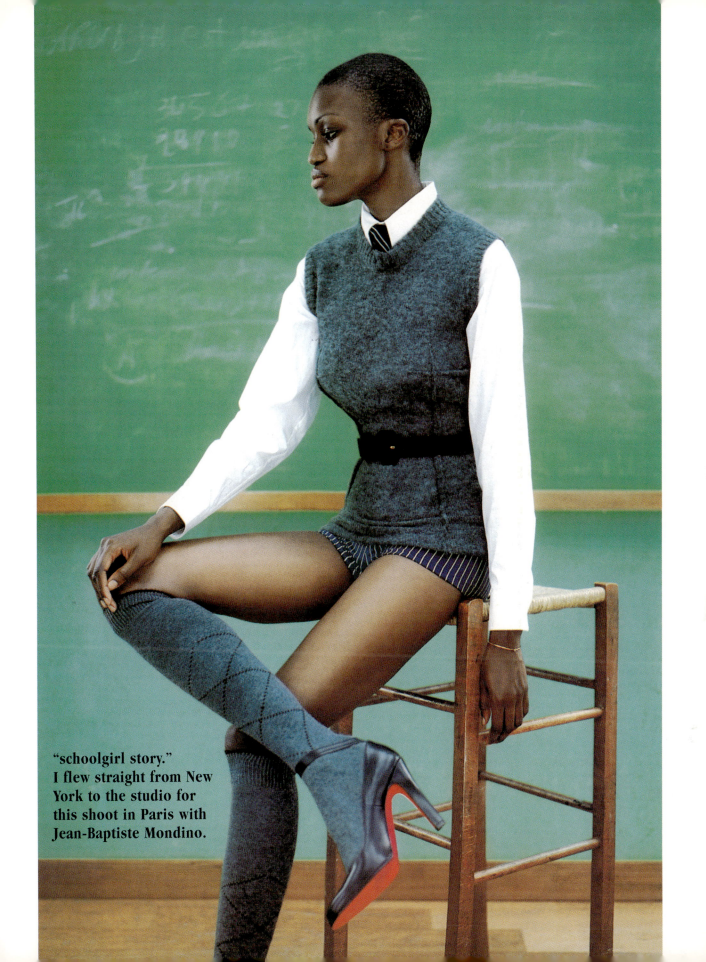

"schoolgirl story."
I flew straight from New
York to the studio for
this shoot in Paris with
Jean-Baptiste Mondino.

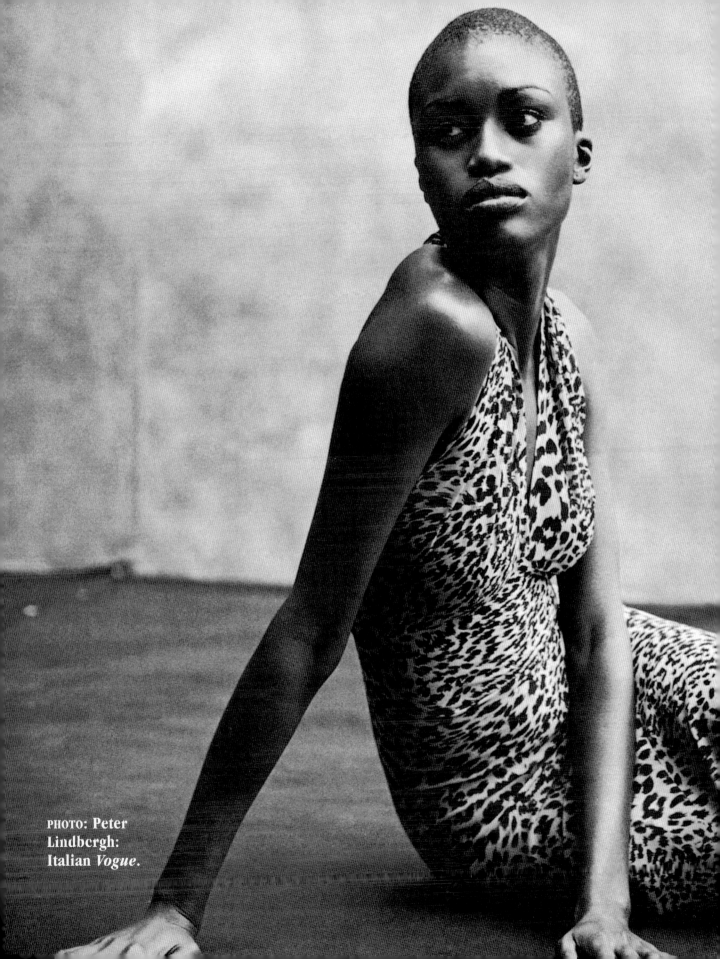

PHOTO: Peter Lindbergh: Italian *Vogue*.

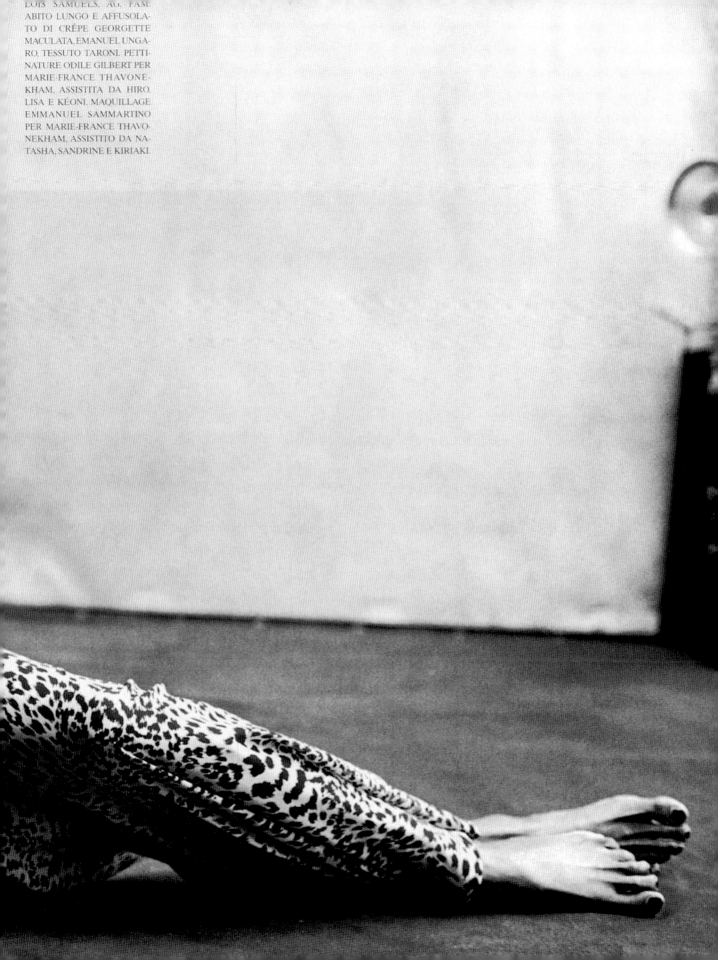

LOIS SAMUELS, AG. FAM.
ABITO LUNGO E AFFUSOLA-
TO DI CRÊPE GEORGETTE
MACULATA, EMANUEL UNGA-
RO, TESSUTO TARONI. PETTI-
NATURE ODILE GILBERT PER
MARIE-FRANCE THAVONE-
KHAM, ASSISTITA DA HIRO,
LISA E KÉONI. MAQUILLAGE
EMMANUEL SAMMARTINO
PER MARIE-FRANCE THAVO-
NEKHAM, ASSISTITO DA NA-
TASHA, SANDRINE E KIRIAKI.

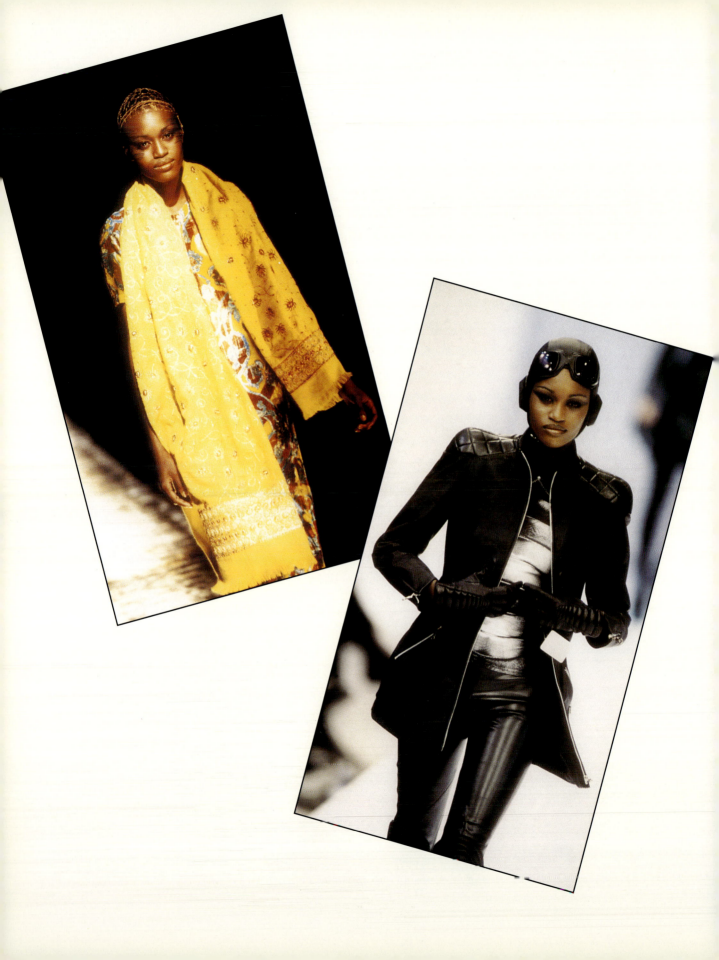

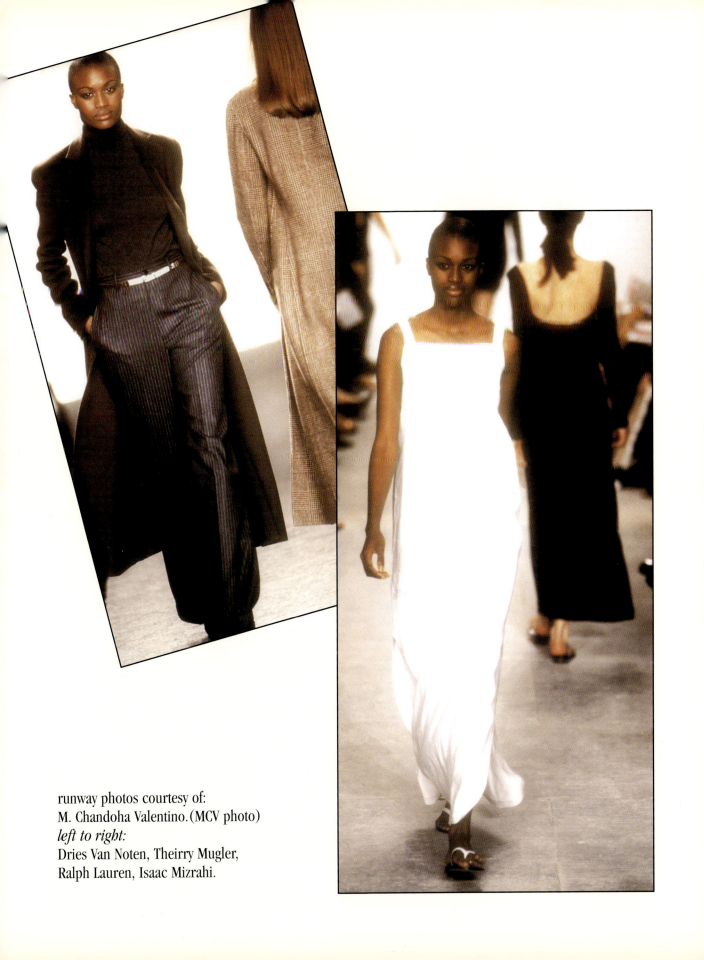

runway photos courtesy of:
M. Chandoha Valentino. (MCV photo)
left to right:
Dries Van Noten, Theirry Mugler,
Ralph Lauren, Isaac Mizrahi.

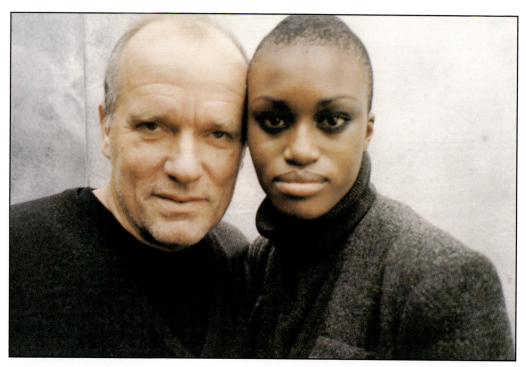

on the set of Italian *Vogue* with
Peter Lindbergh in Paris.

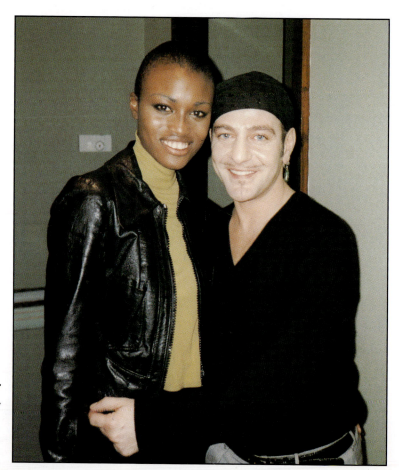

back stage Christian Dior
couture show
with John Galliano.

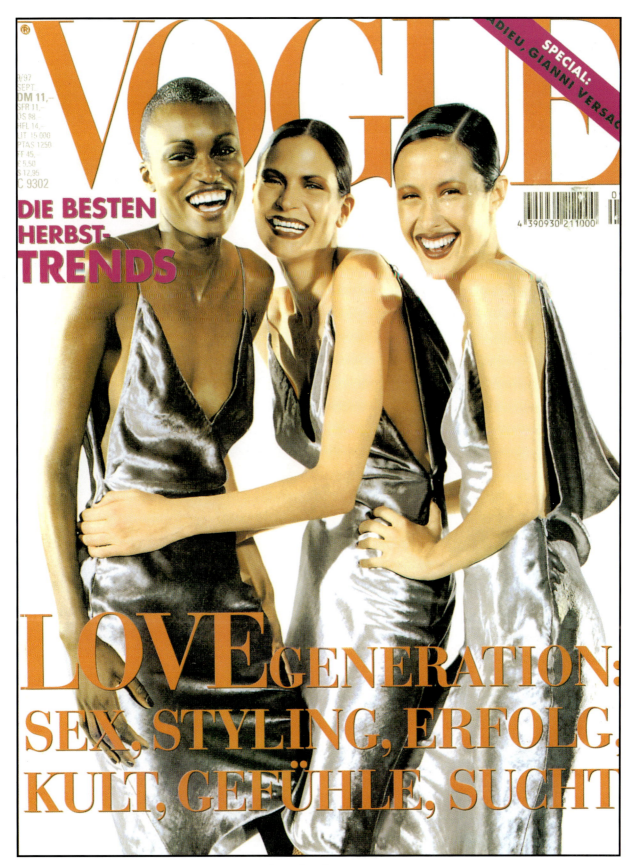

VOGUE

9/97
SEPT.
DM 11,–
SFR 11,–
ÖS 88
HFL 14,–
LIT 15 000
PTAS 1250
FF 45,–
$ 5,50
$ 12,95
C 9302

SPECIAL: ADIEU, GIANNI VERSACE

DIE BESTEN HERBST- TRENDS

4 390930 211000

LOVE GENERATION: SEX, STYLING, ERFOLG. KULT, GEFÜHLE, SUCHT

PHOTO: Walter Chin for German *Vogue.*

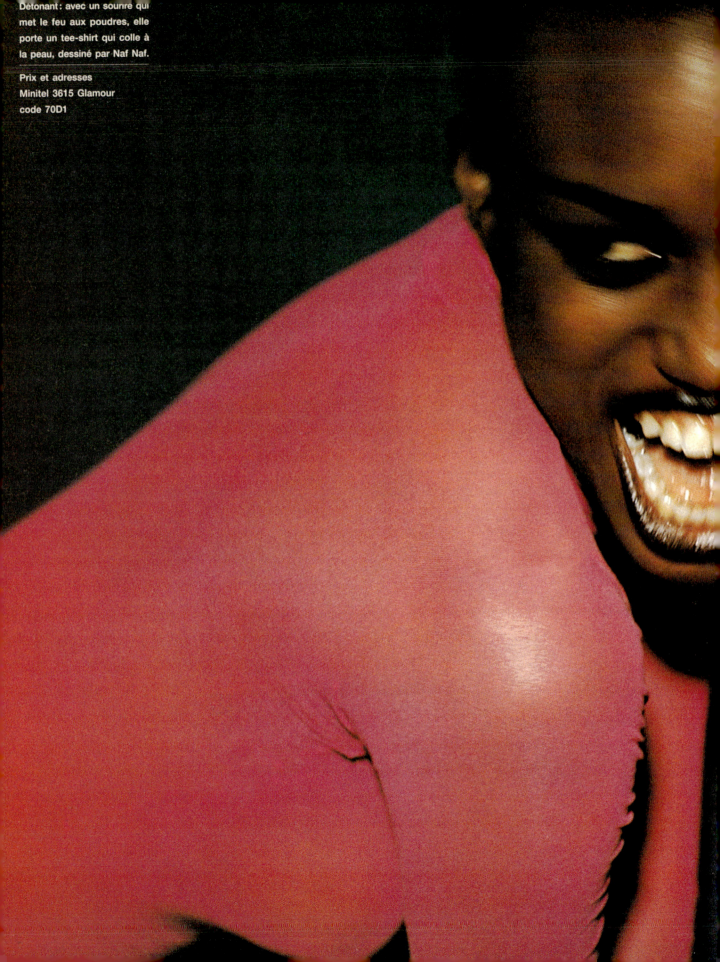

Détonant : avec un sourire qui
met le feu aux poudres, elle
porte un tee-shirt qui colle à
la peau, dessiné par Naf Naf.

Prix et adresses
Minitel 3615 Glamour
code 70D1

My Life as a Model

Real achievement is not all about having fame and making a lot of money. It is also about facing fears and conquering them. It is doing the best at what you want in life to making your dreams come true yet still remaining grounded through it all. There are many roads to be taken in life; some may be beneficial to us and others not. But you have to come through all the hardships in life with dignity, honour and self-respect to become YOU.

I am fully aware that modelling is not a life time career. I am also fully aware that we all are not super-models and we cannot all be supermodels. Equally true is that we cannot all be highly successful. This business is a fickle and unpredictable one that is not as glamorous as it looks, and it demands very, very hard work. For a woman, this business may last 10 to 15 years of her life. Some do it forever; some do not know what else to do while others cross over into other entertainment-related business, as actresses or hosts for television programmes, since image is the number one seller. For a model like myself, being of colour and from an island with very little history in the fashion industry, I would have to carve out my own path.

Entering the fashion industry at an early age is quite beneficial as momentum to build a modelling career. Agencies and their clients prefer to begin working with girls, when they are between the ages of thirteen to fifteen. Personally I find this wrong, as at this tender age they have not discovered themselves as yet. I recommend a good time to begin is after completing high school education, between the ages of seventeen and nineteen.

Again persistence is vital in the business, and it takes tremendous effort to keep going. If you have decided this is what you want to do, you have to be focused on it. You have to dedicate yourself to it as there are thousands of girls entering the market everyday. The apparent glamour may be all enticing but it is best to keep in mind these realities:

- You have to face and deal with insecurities.
- Travel and work can be tiring and stressful. Put yourself first and take care of your health.
- Be of substance so that you do not fall into the world of fantasy.

In today's entertainment-related business, as in the past, drugs present a serious problem which one will certainly have to confront. The pressure of having always to be in the spotlight and always looking good, no matter what the circumstances, may lead some to believe that they need help from substances to give them a boost. This is a big mistake..

Never allow peer pressure to lead you down a path of destruction. I have seen models doing drugs backstage before going on the runway, under the misguided but often proferred belief that it makes them more relaxed or something. Ever so often we hear and read of models who had to check themselves into rehabilitation centres to kick their habits. It is not a pretty thing, drug addiction, so if you can, it is wise to avoid getting into this situation. I will never forget a Couture show I did once for a designer in Paris. A few minutes before the show was about to begin, one of the top models of that moment, arrived very late. She looked pale and almost blue and every muscle in her body was shaking, shaking so uncontrollably, she could not put her clothes or her shoes on as she was so weak. But as usual, the show must go on, she was sent on the runway swaying out of control. She had to be lifted up and carried around to change for the only two outfits she could do, before they released her, as she could not finish the show. I am sure she was paid for that job as once a model is booked for something, and shows up, she must be paid. I was shocked. I had never before experienced anything like this in any of my shows in Jamaica.

We Jamaicans are brought up in an environment that is insular and thus not universal in outlook. Our customs, traditions, way of life are passed on from generation to generation without too much fuss. Thus, when we are thrown into the ocean of life to figure things out for ourselves it can be a horrific experience. You have to be prepared to fight loneliness, poverty, prejudice and the principalities of dark forces when you work in foreign countries and cities.

I used to tell my mother, 'I leave from nothing, and I come back to nothing'. Yes I knew there was the ever omnipresence of God, who was in me and around me, who gave me strength and who worked numerous miracles for me. He must have seen that I needed the miracle of a companion. Indeed loneliness was like a burden, even though I dealt with so many people daily. I guess with my temperament, I preferred at the end of the day to be by myself, rather than trying to know someone new. Travelling, being in different hotels, being always ready to go on shoots, staying in various apartments, makes your life feel so empty especially when you have no one to share your joy or your pain, your success or your failures, your highs or your lows with. After a while parents are not the ones you always get comfort from confiding in. You need something more. It took me a while before I found someone to share my life with, and when this happened. the sisters of the sun shone. Despite the differences in our age, our race and our culture (he is Russian), we are very compatible. There is no feeling as great as the feeling you get when you have someone in your corner. And it is even better when this person has similar

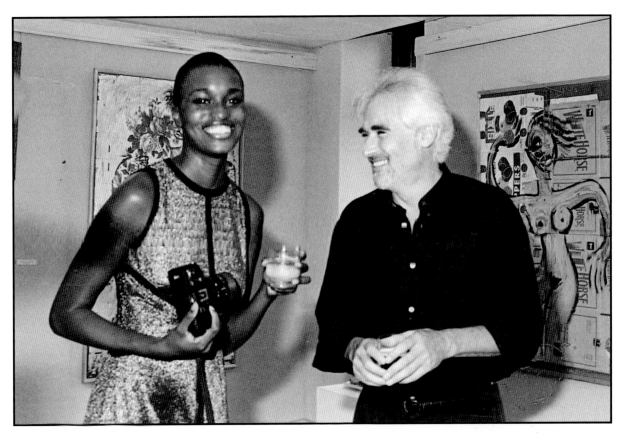

with Alexander at his exhibition at the Museum of Modern Art in Belarus.

interests as you. I consider myself lucky for we both love simplicity, we both love achievements, we both are creative (he is an artist and a writer) and we both see what roles we play in life. Whether you are failing or winning when you find someone special in your corner, nothing matters, once you have each other. It is always nice to return to my Russian warmth and solace.

As models, we have to be ever so careful. I have seen so many girls lose their souls because of their love of material things. Many wealthy men 'love' stunningly attractive women. They take a model shopping, buy her expensive jewelry, show her around the world, give her money and they know they can have her. In reality, these rich men have bought a commodity—the model. So many girls get hooked on to what they can see rather than what they can feel. Yes, we are free to make our choices but at the end of the day what satisfaction do you get when you finally wake up and cannot even smell the fresh air? It is always good to have a shoulder to lean on, but never rush into things. Do not allow yourself to be seen as an object. Take your time to know someone. Many people have their own image of models, and preconceived ones at that.

Personally, in times of loneliness and hardships, I drew strength from the bible and those Sunday morning sermons. Verses 1-2 from Romans, Chapter 10 were especially comforting and helpful:

1.   I beseech you therefore, by the mercies of God, that you present your bodies a living sacrifice, holy, acceptable unto God, which is your reasonable service.
2.   And be not conformed to this world: but be transformed by the renewing of your mind, that you may prove what is good and acceptable and perfect will of God.

Loneliness can be as painful as hunger, but with spiritual food one can always be filled. I remember when I was alone, I got to the point where I was fed up with eating alone in restaurants and cooking for myself, so much so, that at times I lost my appetite all together. So I do know what hunger is.

Negative energy coming from jealousy, greed, prejudice, competitiveness and anger, encircle us in life. This is, however, more prevalent in the modelling world. But:

. . . wait patiently, fret not thyself because of him who prospereth in his way . . . (Psalm 37 vs.7)

I believe it is the will of God for one to acquire certain things, but not everything. I believe it is the will of one to make something of oneself. Oneness with a Supreme Being or Divine Force will certainly provide the spiritual guidance for keeping one's soul intact and one's aspirations in perspective.

Getting the Agency

Some models get lucky and skip the whole process of trying to get an agency. They may have been spotted by an agency scout on the lookout for girls with modelling potential. That was how, I was 'discovered' by Pulse. Having experienced the ups and downs of a modelling career, I deeply feel the need to help aspiring models, now that I am in a position to do so. Here I am offering some useful hints for those trying to get agencies to represent them.

On the first visit to the agency, you should take at least two pictures, one showing the face—a beauty shot, and the other of the body, perhaps wearing a bathing suit, so the body can be seen. Do not put the horse before the cart and incur unnecessary expenses prior to seeing agencies, by renting a photo studio and photographer to take pictures. My Dad did this for me before I left on my first trip with the group from Pulse to Europe and America. He rented a studio in Kingston and also took me on location in Beverly Hills to the home of his associate where a photographer worked for an entire day, taking pictures which were not of international standard. So even though he went afterwards and got a beautiful portfolio for which I could carry them, all this proved to be quite expensive and unessential. I am ever grateful for my Dad's attempts to help me in this way. But the standards of the international market are high, and some things like fashion photography is thus best left to professionals.

The least you have to represent yourself at this initial stage, the better it is, as it leaves open what the agencies believe you are capable of doing.

Before visiting the agency it is very important that you call to make an appointment as different agencies have various requirements regarding age or height of the person. They may also have specific days and hours in which they see models. I also believe that it is good to keep an ear open for modelling competitions. Many agencies all over the world have an annual model competition, and from these, girls are chosen to join their agency.

Once an agency has an interest in you, a contract would usually be offered. (Some agencies do not give contracts, as this allows both models and agency more freedom). Generally this contract lasts for two to three years, and renews itself automatically (that is, if it is not terminated by the model). It is imperative that everything is read and understood before it is signed. This business can be very exploitative so to fully understand the conditions of your contract, get advice from a lawyer or a more experienced person. I believe parents or a guardian of some sort should play a role in the business transactions of the model, to protect the model's interests. Most models, being teenagers are not at all versed in the intricasies of such transactions and may be taken advantage of otherwise. I also believe this approach leads agents to give more attention to the model.

For me, it was difficult to get adjusted in this business. I hated paper work, I hated going through documents and I hated doing the accounting. I just wanted to have enough money to live and be happy. I still have no pleasure in the business and administrative aspects but fashion modelling is a business, and like any business you have to keep track of all transactions.

If you have no one to help you with your contract, it never hurts to ask questions.

If all goes well, you are finally on your way.

then you
are as the kite
you are boundless
for you have no longer a pilot
the master for direction lies within you
led by the elements of the wind and the rain
till at rest

.   .   .

Image

Crucial to a model is the image she has to project everyday of her professional life. Apart from being tall and skinny, there were other important things I had to keep in mind like the condition of my skin.

Having a blemish-free skin free from any significant scars or pimples is important. I am one of those lucky persons, who do not have to deal with facial breakouts. But if you happen to suffer from this, make special effort to always cleanse your skin after a long day and never go to bed without removing makeup. Even if you do not wear makeup, the air can be very polluted, so cleansing is essential. Once in a while I would steam my face over some boiling water as this helps to unclog the pores. The worst that has ever happened to my skin happened in the April of 1998. Thank God it was a slow period in my professional life. I thought I was in the middle of a plague. I just remember being extremely weak and sick. There were strange bumps coming up all over my body; lumps in the back of my neck and boils in my head. I could not move and was in bed with a high fever. I never go to the doctor, if anything is wrong with me, God the greatest physician will fix it. That has always been my philosophy, as far as I am concerned. Foreign doctors are always making things seem more serious than they really are, and charging more than they really should. Anyway, my companion insisted I go to the hospital, where I was told I had chicken pox. My skin was a disaster, not to mention my face. In this predicament, I discovered that nothing beats Palmers Cocoa Butter Formula, and Aveenos Bath Powder.

Another important asset every model should take care of is the teeth. Take care of your teeth. It is easier and cheaper to take care of them on an everyday basis, than having to deal with the dentists' bills in the long run. Thank God for St. Elizabeth hard sugar cane, my teeth can tackle anything, but try to avoid sugar candies, like the coconut grater cakes I used to devour, that did send me to the dentist many a time.

As a lean physique is a prerequisite, being over weight may pose a problem. Again I am lucky with the genes that run in the family. I can eat as much as I want, as I get so much pleasure in eating good foods. Nevertheless, if you have weight problem, do not starve yourself to remain slender, or take any unnecessary harmful action, to achieve and maintain a certain body weight. Forget those diet pills, cosmetic

PHOTO: **Ruven Afanador**
for *Scene* Magazine.

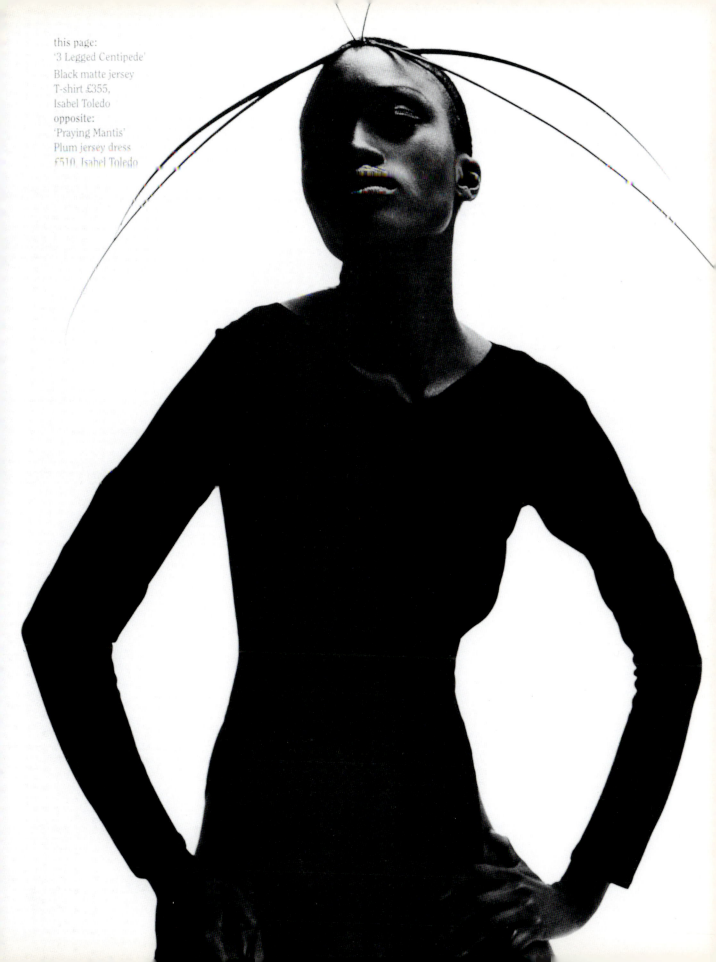

this page:
'3 Legged Centipede'
Black matte jersey
T-shirt £355,
Isabel Toledo
opposite:
'Praying Mantis'
Plum jersey dress
£510, Isabel Toledo

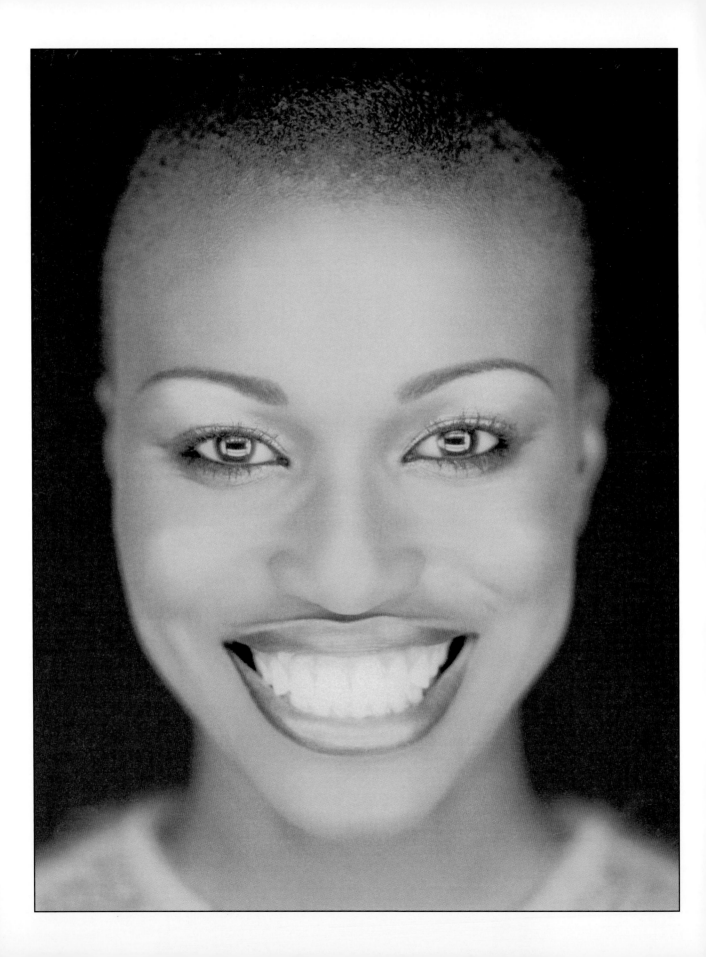

surgeries and drugs, as it is not worth dying to lose a couple of pounds. Ever so often you hear of young women, losing their lives through such hazardous means. There are some simple yet effective ways to lose and maintain weight. Cut back on eating foods with too much carbohydrates and sweets. Try exercising, maybe going to the gym, swimming and doing aerobics may help. Keeping to this regimen, however, requires some discipline. I do some stretching exercises, which you will see further in the book.

The required height for models starts from around 5 feet 9 inches. But in recent times, height seems a bit insignificant as quite a few established models, (for example Kate Moss) have been under the recommended height. Yet again being tall does not dictate everything. I remember when I just began modelling internationally. I was very shy and insecure, so my body language was very poor, until I built up some confidence. It is hard to say you will not be shy but be alert to what comes across to your clients. Try to sit up straight, and walk like a lady. For having 'presence' works favourably. Being conventionally pretty is not synonymous with having 'presence' . . . but the way in which you carry yourself and attain your respect does. If you have some dance training, like I had in ballet in my schooldays, you will understand 'presence' better. It is akin to what dancers term 'pull up' and a certain carriage of oneself and has nothing to do with just being good-looking. This certainly explains the success of many internationally-acclaimed models society at large consider 'ugly'.

. . . see my beautiful smile?

PHOTO: Robert Trachenberg.

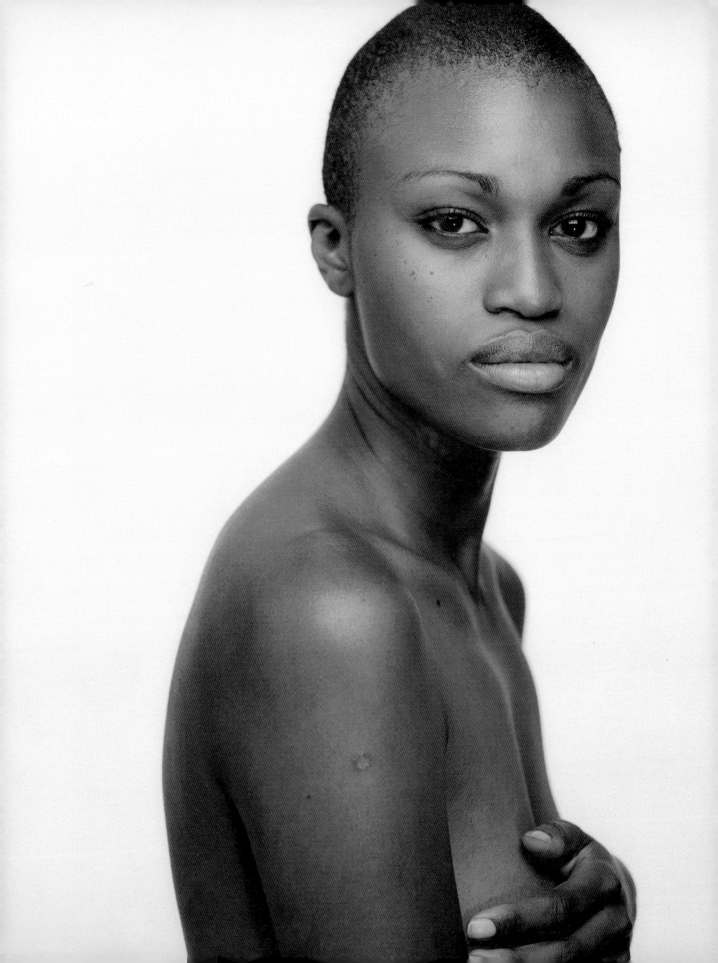

'Garbage in —garbage out'
'You are what you eat— You look like you think'

Since beauty is the issue here, the body should be treated with utmost care.

Proper food should be eaten, exercise should be taken in moderation and the body should not be mistreated in any way. It is very hard for me to maintain a healthy and stable diet in this business, as I was constantly travelling with sometimes all of my possessions in two suitcases, hopping from plane to train, to taxi. Away from home, I did not have a mother or father, to see to it that I was eating properly. I have this problem where I would forget to eat, sometimes because of anxiety, trying to keep ahead of time or sometimes I just simply forget that I should eat. There is this drive, this urge that makes food less important than what I need to achieve in a day. Sometimes I was just picky, and in turn I would be weak and dizzy and unable to go through the day. To avoid this, I encourage all models to always carry fruits, water and crackers with them when travelling. You may sometimes have problems adjusting to the foods of different countries, so it is good to always have your supply of what you are accustomed to until you get in sync with theirs. I remember the first time I spent one month in Paris. I suffered from terrible stomach problems, as I could not get adjusted to their foods. At that time I had stopped eating meats; I lived on cheese sandwiches so much, till I could not stand the sight of another baguette. I try to be a vegetarian everywhere else but in Jamaica where the temptation to tuck in to home cuisine is too irresistable.

When you do not eat properly, the body becomes vulnerable and very susceptible to illness. I was very lucky not to be ill, but even if I were and knew I should probably see a doctor, my faith would heal me before anything got out of hand.

You have to learn how to discipline yourself, and to make it a part of your routine to take vitamin tablets, especially vitamin C (if you are not eating at the right times), drink lots of water, eat fruits and vegetables (preferably uncooked ones) and avoid too much sweet and oily foods. Also it is very important to get good rest. Instead of being on the scene and partying all night, drinking too much alcohol in a cloud of smoke, pamper yourself with long relaxing baths and rest. Good rest benefits the skin.

A deep belief of mine for good health and radiant beauty is having good thoughts, and having a good

PHOTO: **Marc Baptiste.**

heart. With my spiritual belief, I am able to avoid harbouring negative thoughts. I see no necessity for envying, hating or being jealous of other people as it does not help me nor change anything.

In this business, where unhealthy competition is rampant there is a great tendency to find girls hating one another all out of jealousy. Jealousy and hate make people ugly and this negativism is reflected in their personality.

Believing you are better than the other person because of some physical, social or spiritual reason makes you ugly. So does gossiping and spreading rumours about people to make them look bad, so you may look good.

Be positive and turn all negatives into positive. Maybe there is a lesson in life you need to learn to enhance your personal growth as a person. But if you fight negative with negative it only make matters worse. Avoid being one of the thousands in this business who wear masks to cover their hypocritical, envious and untruthful ways because neither plastic surgery nor makeup can fix that ugliness.

Plastic surgery is so readily available today that many girls are resorting to it. I personally find it amusing when I see girls change right before my eyes. I remember two girls who had their breasts enlarged the old-fashioned way. Instead of having the insertion in the nipples or through the armpits which is quite expensive, they had those ugly surgical scars underneath the breasts which were very visible. Obviously proper healing did not take place as they had expected. I remember them being so embarrassed when it was time to change backstage at the shows. They had no freedom. I also noticed some girls who started in the business with square noses, ended up with real triangular ones shortly after. They were lucky to come out alive, and in good condition, from under the surgeons' knife. I see it this way: we are free to do whatever we choose, but we must learn to accept and love ourselves the way we are, and remember that *'real beauty comes from within'.*

hyprocrites

you share your laughter
with the glimmer in your eyes
but the darkness of your skin
doesn't hide what's within
you share your joy
with smiles so wide to touch your ear
but the whiteness of your skin
doesn't hide who's within
a spark of anger sets the fire
a flint of envy
corrupts your everything
a flower with a weed
and land without seeds
that's all to see
the bitter sweet taste
this beautiful ugliness
is you

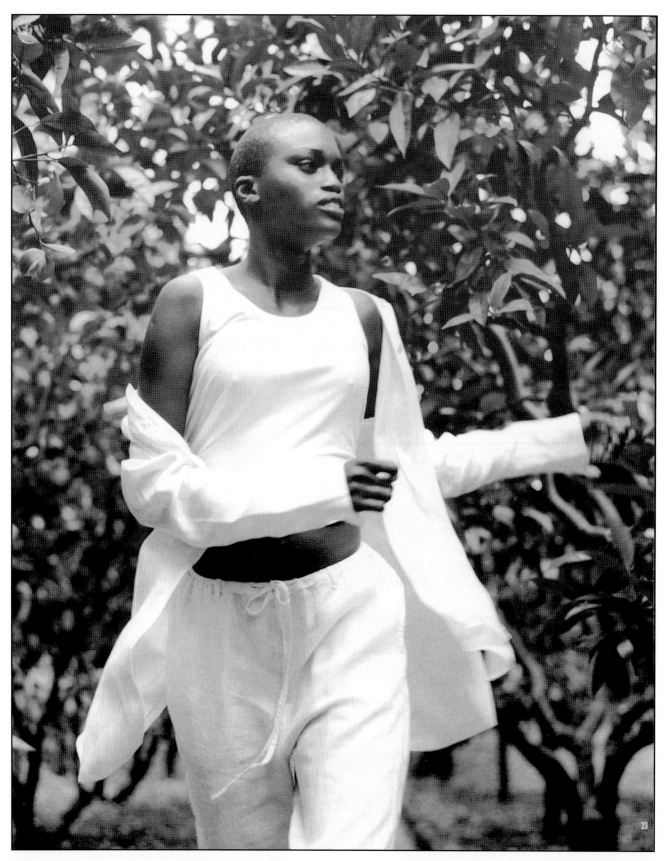

jogging for Oilily advertising in Sante Stefano, Tuscany.

Exercise

As is a golden rule, exercise is perhaps the model's best friend.

A type of exercise should be chosen. Walking is unavoidable, and it is the most convenient method of getting around on castings and also just the best way to discover and know your way around any city. I did a lot of walking in the beginning of my career, mainly because I had no money to be taking a taxi, and I had to save the little I had, by not taking the subway too often. Sometimes the amount of walking I did in one day was enough exercise to last one, an entire month.

It is beneficial for models to exercise at least three times a week to keep in shape and to develop fully-toned muscles. Joining gyms and yoga centres in any country is quite easy without having to spend much money. I did yoga, which is a Hindu system of relaxation, exercise and meditation, controlling the body and mind. It is a low paced kind of exercise, but very demanding. Knowing me I did it only for a short while as I had to get out of the routine. Then again, I was born lucky with my body weight and apart from all the walking and the biking I did in New York and Amsterdam, I never really saw the necessity for additional exercise. Going to the gym, for me, would only be a burden to think about.

Jogging, I occasionally did along the Hudson River, but I feel that jogging only drags the body down, even though it is a really good way to just burn up a sweat.

What I did do and still do, (which I have illustrated), are stretching exercises. These exercises keep the body's energy flowing. So if I feel a little stiff, like from travelling and not moving around for a while, to keep the energy flowing, I do these simple exercises.

Whether one is a little overweight or slender, it pays to remember that exercise is beneficial. Starving, diet pills, heavy smoking or drug taking are pathetic methods of maintaining body weight and in the long run, could be very destructive to your health, your self esteem and your career.

1. Lung and large intestine meridian stretch:
With your feet shoulder width apart, hook thumbs behind your back and stretch fingers outwards. As you breathe out, bend forward keeping arms straight. The feeling should be of an enjoyable stretch. Make sure you are not tensing up and breathe slowly for at least a minute.

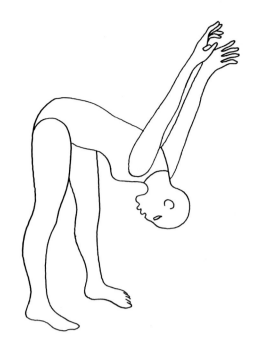

2. Spleen and stomach meridian stretch:
Sit with your knees bent outwards and rest on your elbows. Breathe slowly and as you get more comfortable stretch further until you are able to put both arms above your head. If you have discomfort or pain in your lower back, go back to the first position.

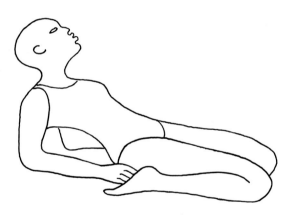

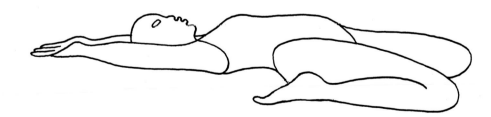

3. Kidney and bladder meridian stretch

With your legs straight out in front of you, bend forwards from the hips and reach your hands as far down the legs as you can comfortably go.

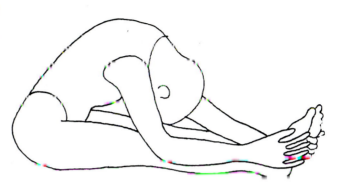

4. Liver and gall bladder meridian stretch
Spread your legs as wide as you can. While keeping them straight bend from the waist and stretch.

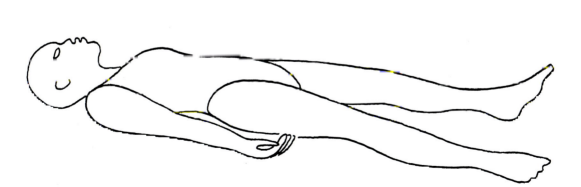

5. Be sure to keep breathing slowly for all these exercises, and lay flat on the back after all is done.

The Face

A model's face can be her fortune or misfortune; so meticulous care is essential to ensure that she always or nearly always becomes 'the face that launched a thousand ships'.

It all boils down to the face. If the body looks good and the clothes fit perfectly and the face is a mess —forget the rest. Proper care must be taken with the face.

First and foremost, eyebrows must be tweezed at least twice per week. Sometimes models get lazy and prefer waiting for the makeup artist to clean up our brows on the job. But to save time, always be prepared. If you grow a little moustache, (as you know some women do), always use a removal cream such as Nair, to get rid of it, or get a wax done. It is not too appealing when all the visible signs of your male hormones are evident on your face.

Secondly, if you are not used to the sun, stay in the shade, and be wrinkle free for many years. If you decide to sit in the sun and have great fun remember your sun block cream. Being Jamaican, I love the sun. I really do not see the necessity in wearing sun block cream; if I do, it is because I do not want to disappear in the dark. But if you are fair in complexion, you are well advised to use sun block cream or sunscreen to prevent skin damage due to both the UVA and UVB elements of sunlight.

Smoking is no good for the skin, and no good for your health or the health of the people around you. If you do not smoke refrain from starting as it is a tough habit to break.

Sleep is essential for good skin. Whenever one lacks sleep, the skin tends to look real blotchy and the eyes bloody.

You should never forget to cleanse and moisturize your face. You need to have a clean face before you can apply makeup. And drink plenty of water to hydrate yourself and your skin.

PHOTO: Matthew Jordon Smith
MAKEUP: Roxanne Floyd
On the set of *Essence.*

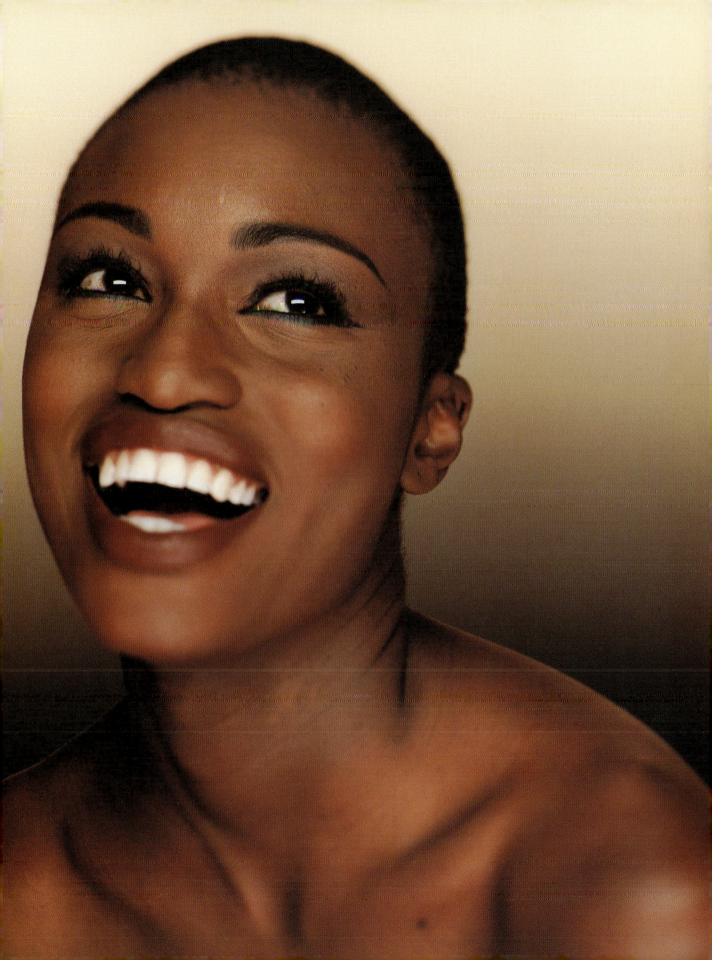

Makeup

*M*akeup only looks good if the skin looks good. We have already discussed the essentials for good-looking skin. Sleep, being a non-smoker, drinking a substantial amount of water, cleansing of the skin and moisturizing are steps which should be religiously followed.

Whether you consider yourself beautiful or not, makeup plays a role in enhancing the facial features of a woman, even though there is a saying 'attitude does more than makeup'.

Personally I go for the natural look as I really do not fancy the makeup stuff. But as a professional model, I am compelled to use makeup when on the job. In applying makeup there are some simple steps I usually follow.

Steps to be taken before applying your makeup:
- Make sure your face is properly cleansed.
- If you have dry skin be sure to moisturize; I sometimes use olive oil or Lancome's hydration moisturizer.
- If your skin is oily to avoid over-hydration blot away excess moisturizers with a piece of tissue as excess moisture only prevents makeup from holding.
- Make sure the foundation being used matches your skin type.
  (do not check colour match on the hand, but on the face)
- Make sure your eyebrows are properly groomed; beautiful makeup does not look good when brows need a tweeze.

I believe a woman should not apply doses of makeup to her face. It is not attractive, and there is no need to have other people believing that she has to use a chisel when removing it. People who have blemished skin or birth marks on their faces, tend to do this, and even some people with beautiful skin, but my advice to you is your imperfection can be your beauty, and even more so when you accept it. The lighter the make up the better it is, as it remains fresh for the entire day and it does not crack cach time you try to smile.

Steps to take when applying simple makeup:

• Foundation if needed, should be applied to the areas that needs the most, for example under and around the eyes and around the lips. It should be applied evenly so there is no blotching.

• Foundation should be applied with fingers or a damp sponge. Personally I prefer using my fingertips as it goes on more evenly.

• Apply makeup in a 'true to life' light especially if you are going out on appointments.

• It is best to apply eye shadows if needed after applying foundation.

• Dust face lightly with powder when finished, and contour with a blush. In case you do not have a blush, lipstick or some lip balm can be used for the same purpose, if blended in with the fingers for contouring.

• Leave the application of mascara for the last.

For models going on castings, the least makeup worn the better it is, unless otherwise requested by the client. Sometimes if models are asked to go on commercial castings, they are requested to use more makeup as it works well with the strong lighting.

All models should have their own makeup bags, to always take on assignments. This will prove extremely handy in case the makeup artists do not have the right colour, or if the model has an allergic reaction to the ones available. I remember on one of my first shows in Milan, Italy. I was the only person of colour in the show, and not one makeup artist offered to do my makeup. It was a terrible let down feeling, but . . . anyway, I hit the runway and glowed naturally.

Overall, for your own peace of mind, always have your own stuff, as you can never predict how your day will go, even if you plan it. That way, you will never be caught unaware.

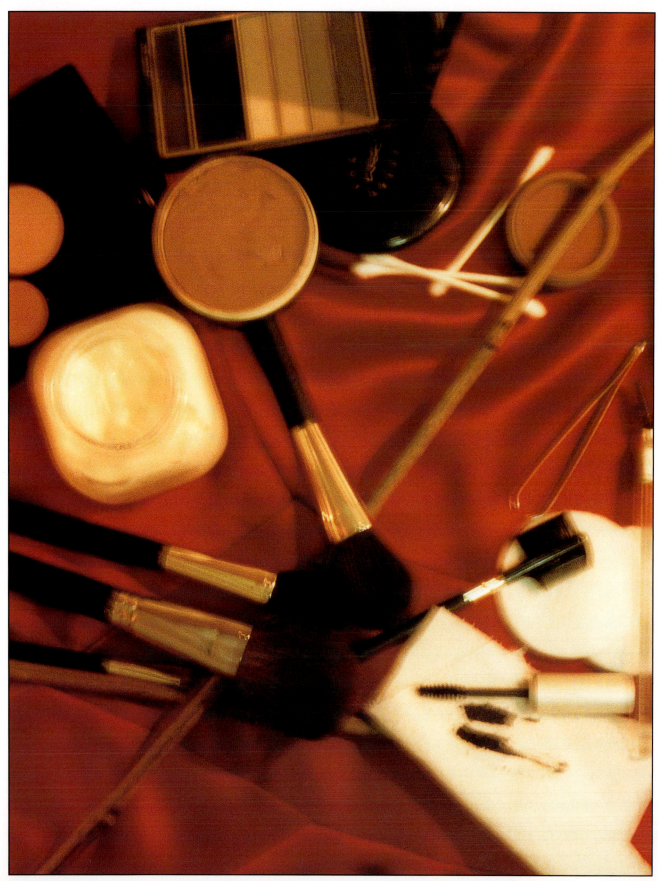

enjoying the sun in Tuscany.

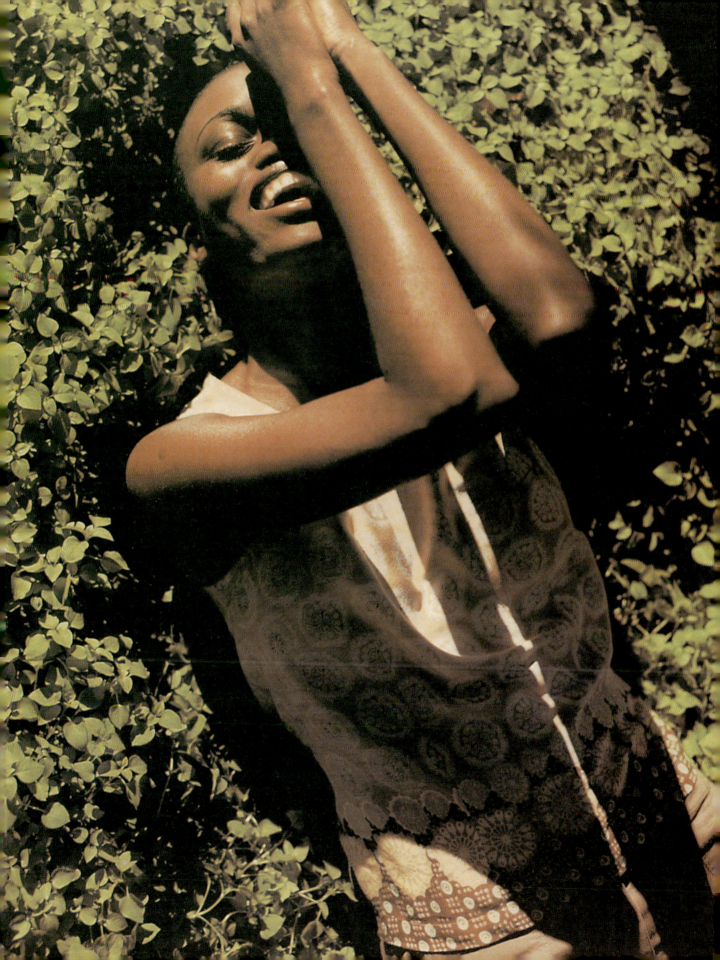

The Removal of Body Hair

In modelling, the sight of any skin area on the body with even a hint of hair is unacceptable, so models are expected to remove all visible hair except (of course) the hair on their heads.

Effective and convenient methods of hair removal:
- *Shaving*

This method of temporary hair removal is the one most used by young women. It takes no time and you just do it while you are having your shower. The only problem I find with this as a black woman is that of ingrown hairs, under the arms and in the pubic areas. Make sure that you shave before going on a job. Growing up in Jamaica, it was not important for a woman to shave her legs; actually the men there do not mind women having unshaved legs. I remember one of my early bookings. I had totally forgotten to shave my legs before going, and I only remember running out to buy a shaver and putting my legs in the wash basin of the bathroom to shave them. It was the most painful bloody thing I have ever done. So be prepared at all times.

- *Waxing*

This is a painful yet very effective method. The hair takes a longer time to grow back, and if it does, it is thinner and therefore less visible.

- *Electrolysis*

   This is the method by which electrical currents are used to destroy the hair roots individually.

- *Removal creams*

These creams, for example, Nair and Neet have chemicals that weaken the hair from the roots making them fall out.

Going on Castings

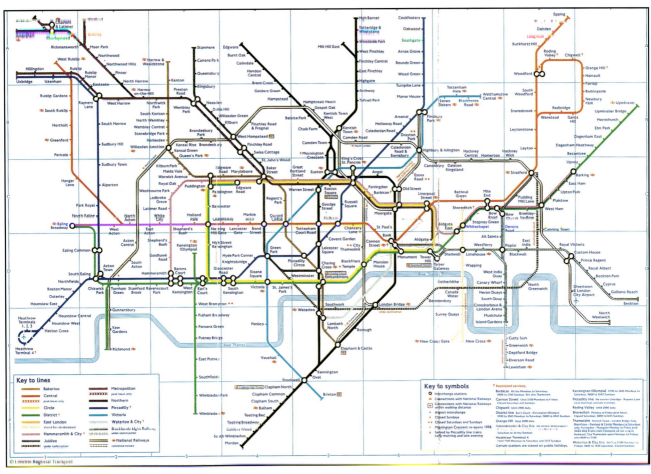

London underground.

*N*ever do as I did when I first came to New York. I remember being so frustrated, spending more time being lost, than being at my appointments. I could not figure out the east from the west of Manhattan! To prevent such mishaps, it is imperative for a model to obtain maps of the city before arrival. Study the underground system of each city, because this is the fastest, cheapest and most effective way to get around.

On arriving in the city, the first thing a model has to do is to go on castings. On these castings, she meets photographers who may be willing to test her in order to build up both her portfolio and his. The portfolio is a book that looks like a photo album which she uses to represent herself. Potential clients can then gauge for themselves the prospects of engaging the model, by looking at her portfolio. While going on these go-sees or castings the model carries a composite in her portfolio, which are cards designed with several of her photographs and her statistics, which she leaves for the clients' files. These cards are also used by the agency for promoting her.

Presentation and approach are very important topics at this level. If you are not dressed or groomed properly, or if your energy or aura is negative due to depression, insecurity or other personal problems, it has an effect in the way you get across to the client. Rejection is ever present and at times very harsh in this business. You have to learn to be strong with optimism not to allow this to affect your behaviour. You have to remember that you cannot be 'the girl' for 'the job' all the time. This business can be seasonal with its choice of image periodically changing. The 'desired' image may be Ethnic one season, Afro the next and Asian to follow.

As I stated before, it took some time for me to land my first job. Sometimes I would go on five to six castings per day for an entire week and not get one job. Yes, it is disappointing, and yes, you do not feel encouraged. You do not know if the problem is you, or it is just a season where your look is not really in. But look on the bright side for the proverbial silver lining; each day you are living and seeing more of the different cities and their varied cultures. And when you continue to believe in yourself, good things will surely come to you.

From going on these castings and getting tested by a few photographers, the next step is doing jobs for clients, as they are now able to see what your capabilities are in front of the camera.

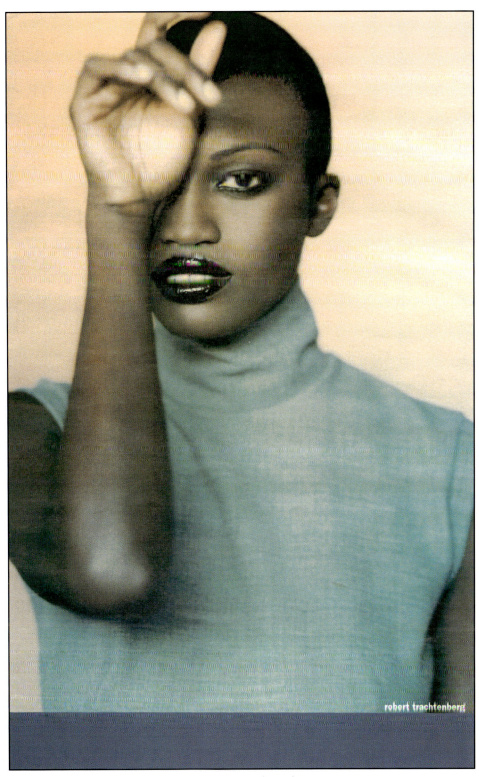

my personal card

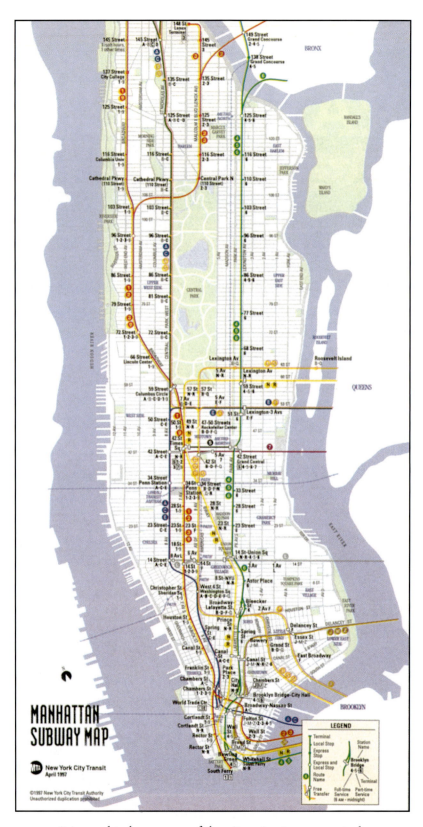

it is good to have maps of the city prior to your arrival,
especially of the subway . . .

On the set

A day of shooting usually lasts from 5-9 hours. The set consists of the photographer, his assistants, the makeup artist, the hairstylist, the stylist of wardrobe, the art director and the model(s). I remember how scared I was the first time on a set. I was shooting a cover try for the American magazine, Essence. I was such a nervous wreck. I will never know how I went through that day. Obviously I failed to get the job. It took me a while to warm up in front of the camera. And it took me an even longer time to warm up in front of an entire crew. Even today at times I still become nervous on the first picture. For me, being the introvert, reading a book or the day's paper relaxes me. But to break the ice talking to the photographer is worth trying, as you will get an understanding of what he expects of you for the shoot. When a kind of affinity is established between the model and the photographer, the end result, the photographs are unbelievably super.

PRIDE

April/May
1996
£1.95 UK

DO CHRISTIAN MEN MAKE BETTER LOVERS?

THE RISE AND RISE OF MONTEL WILLIAMS

WIN A FREE TRIP TO ST LUCIA

COVER GIRL LOIS SAMUELS NEW FACE OF THE 90S

The secret of mind-blowing sex

Irene Cara on the Fame game

Plus hot hair, beauty and fashion tips

ISSN 0963-1720
04
9 770963 172007
Ghana ₵3000 Nigeria N150
SA R2.95 Netherlands Dfl9.95

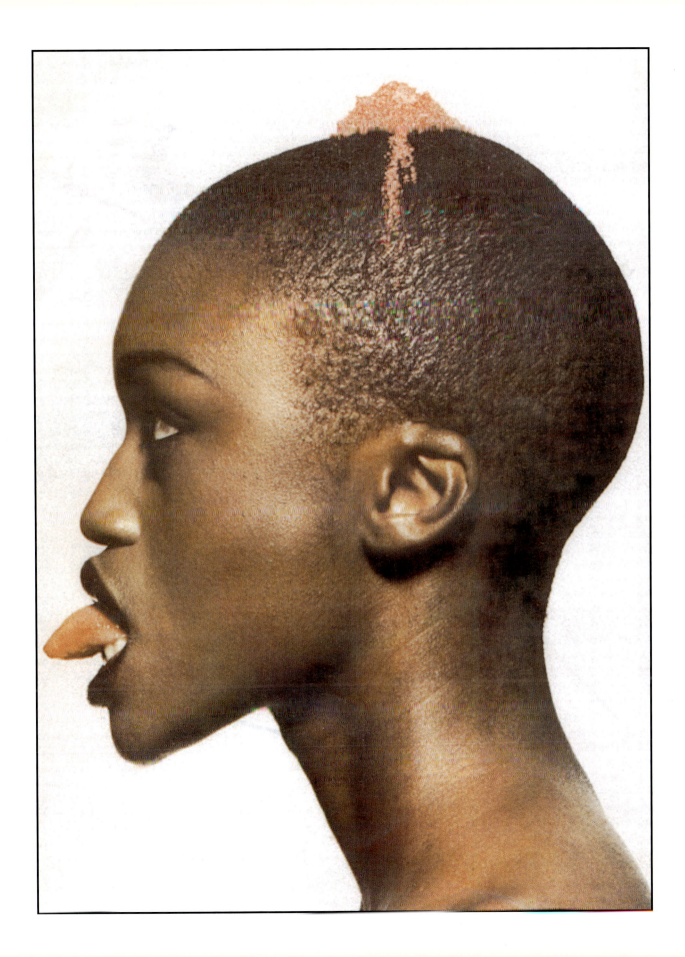

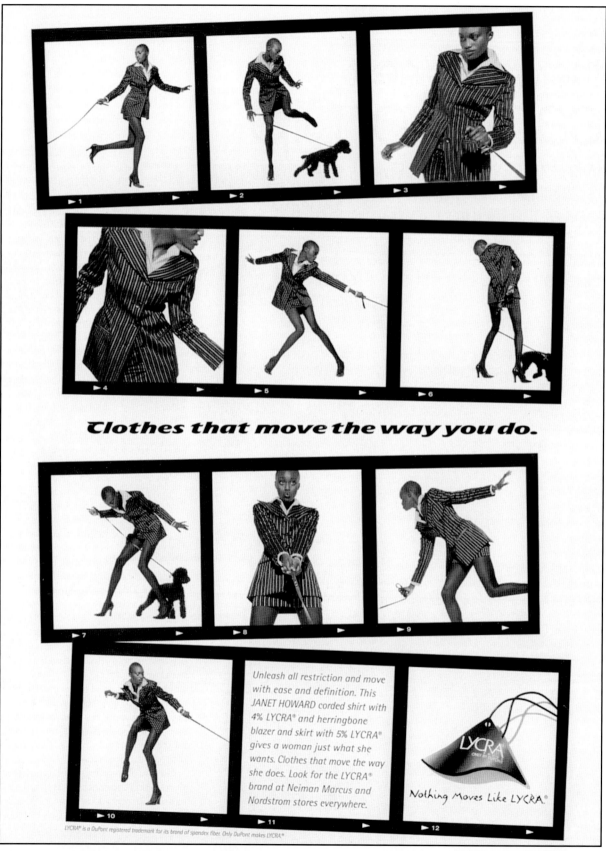

Clothes that move the way you do.

Unleash all restriction and move with ease and definition. This JANET HOWARD corded shirt with 4% LYCRA® and herringbone blazer and skirt with 5% LYCRA® gives a woman just what she wants. Clothes that move the way she does. Look for the LYCRA® brand at Neiman Marcus and Nordstrom stores everywhere.

Nothing Moves Like LYCRA®

LYCRA® is a DuPont registered trademark for its brand of spandex fiber. Only DuPont makes LYCRA®

on set with a poodle.

in Amsterdam shooting Dutch *Elle* with Marcel Vander Vlught.

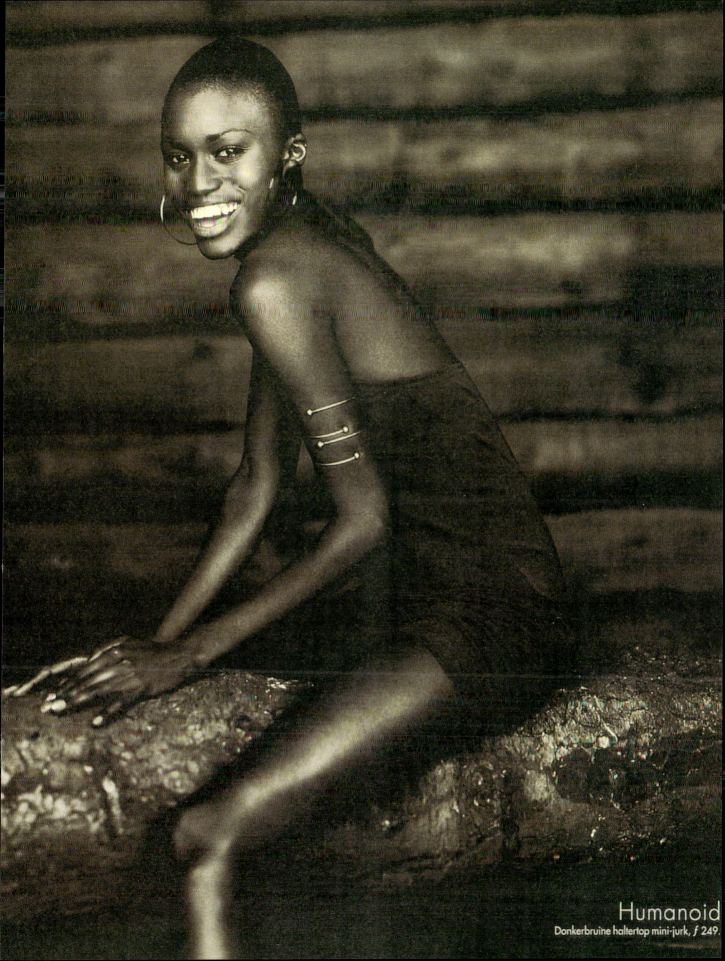

Humanoid
Donkerbruine haltertop mini-jurk, f 249.

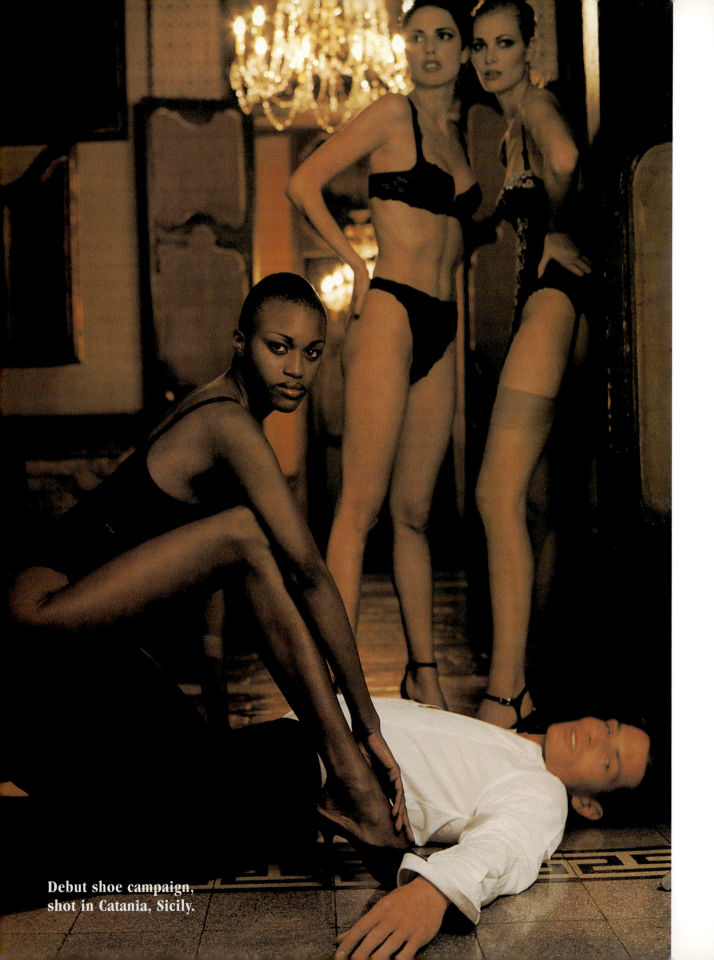

Debut shoe campaign,
shot in Catania, Sicily.

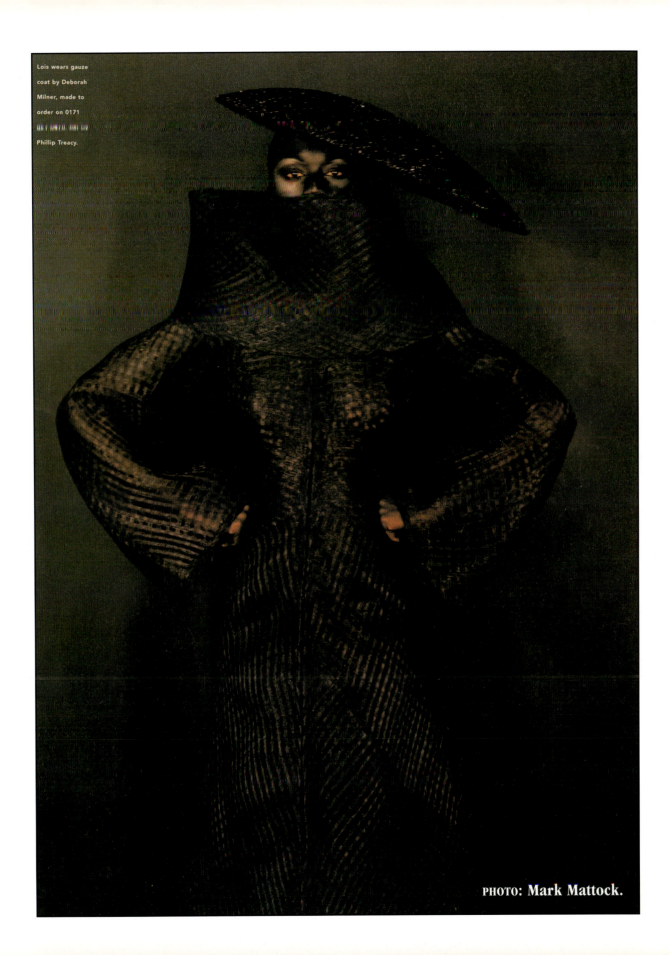

Lois wears gauze
coat by Deborah
Milner, made to
order on 0171

Phillip Treacy.

PHOTO: **Mark Mattock.**

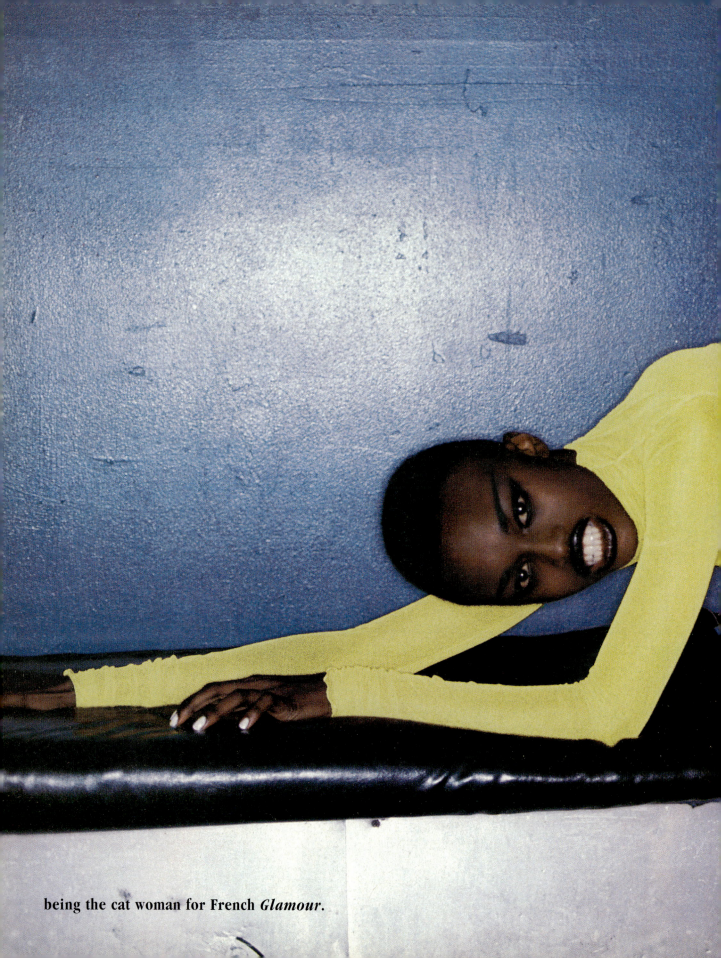

being the cat woman for French *Glamour*.

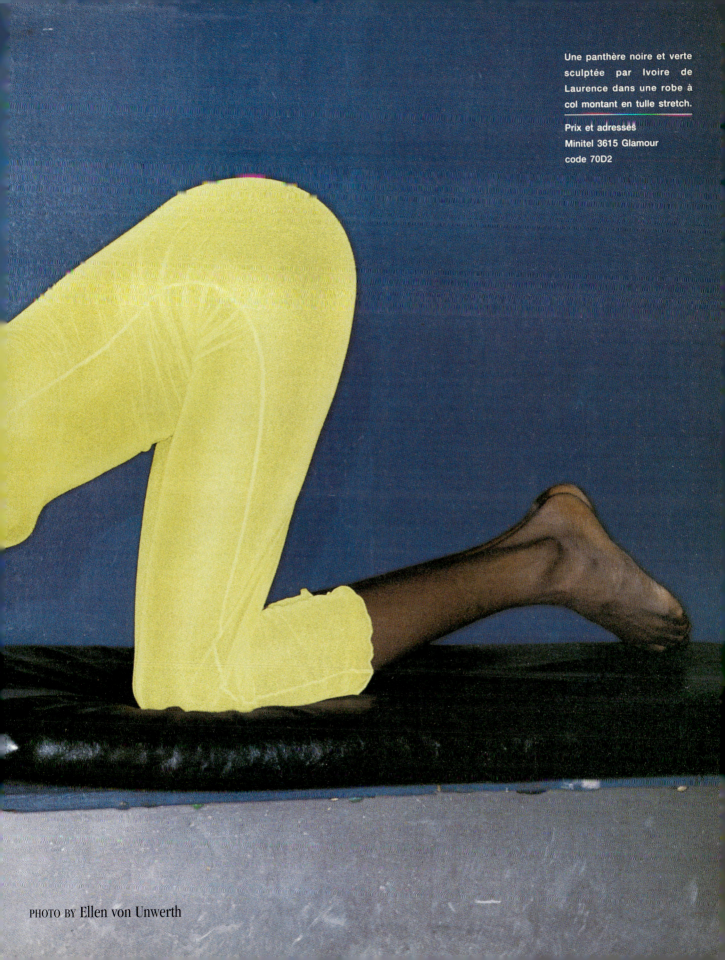

Une panthère noire et verte
sculptée par Ivoire de
Laurence dans une robe à
col montant en tulle stretch.

Prix et adresses
Minitel 3615 Glamour
code 70D2

PHOTO BY Ellen von Unwerth

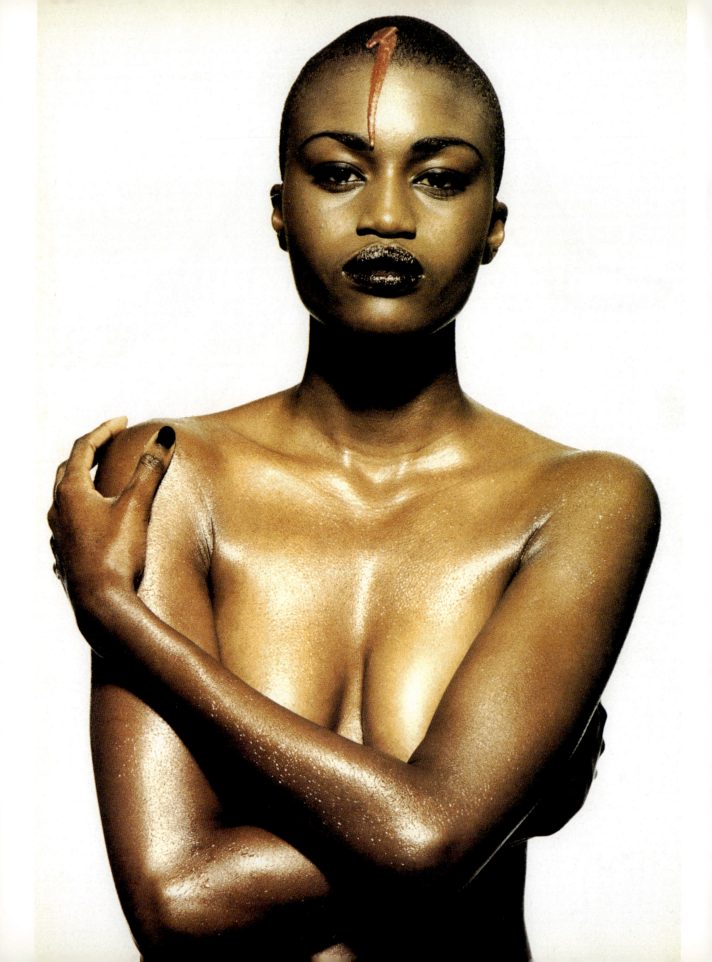

Nudes

Choices dictate everything in life. Being photographed in the nude depends on the model. The model should not allow anyone to force her into doing something she does not want to do or is not comfortable with. The true beauty in a woman's body to me is found inside, but for others it is the physical body itself. The body can be beautiful; it is the way in which the picture is taken, that may make it insulting to the woman.

The line separating true art and pornography is not discernible to many. Pornography insults a woman, no matter how beautiful she is. Art treats the nude form with respect and elevates both model and artist (photographer/painter/sculptor) to a higher realm. Pornography is vulgar while Art is sublime. If a model has the slightest doubt of being photographed nude, then she should heed her own inner voice. Take care that you are not exploited by photographers whose integrity you are unsure of.

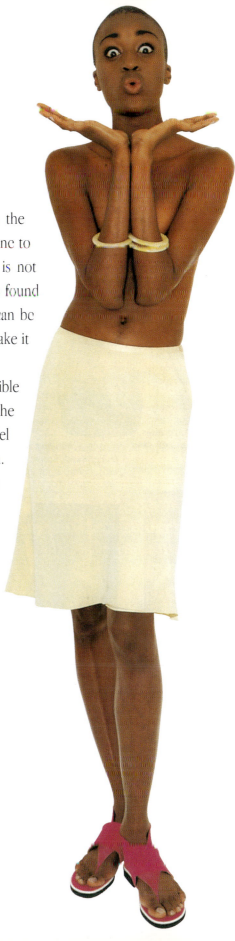

95

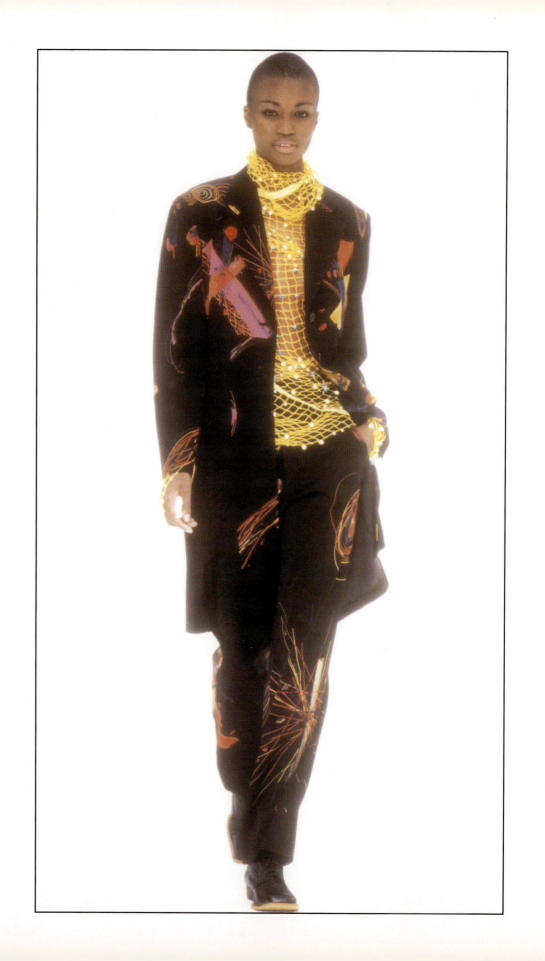

The Runway

This is one aspect of modelling I really enjoy, even though it took me a little while to adapt to it. The presentation of clothes on the international market, was totally different from the technique I had a dapted in Jamaica where unnecessary drama often took place on stage. From the beginning I knew the main reason for having fashion shows was to show the clothes. The model matters, since her presence carries the clothes, but she remains secondary to the designers' creations.

A show rarely exceeds 45 minutes, which is usually 45 minutes of pure energy and excitement. This area of modelling I believe is enjoyed most by models, as they get the opportunity to go out and sashay down the catwalk.

It is hard to tell a model not to be shy or scared when doing a fashion show especially on the first few occasions. I still get butterflies before I get out there, but all I can say is, with time and experience, you grow to become less affected by all the eyes staring at you as you grace the runways. I was lucky not to have fallen like Naomi Campbell did once on the runway which was very funny, but I remember once, while doing a show for Givenchy, I was scared out of my wits wearing circular heeled shoes and red contact lens in my eyes. I could barely see and could barely walk. That was certainly a trauma. But that is perhaps the fun of it all.

at the Louvre in Paris showing
the clothes for Issey Miyake,
one of my favourite designers.

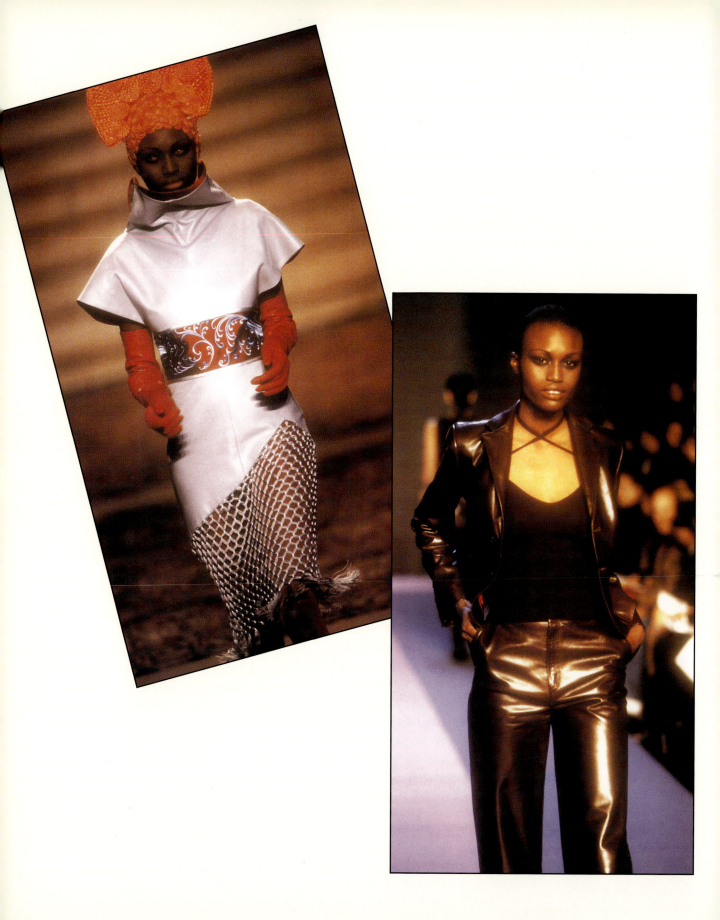

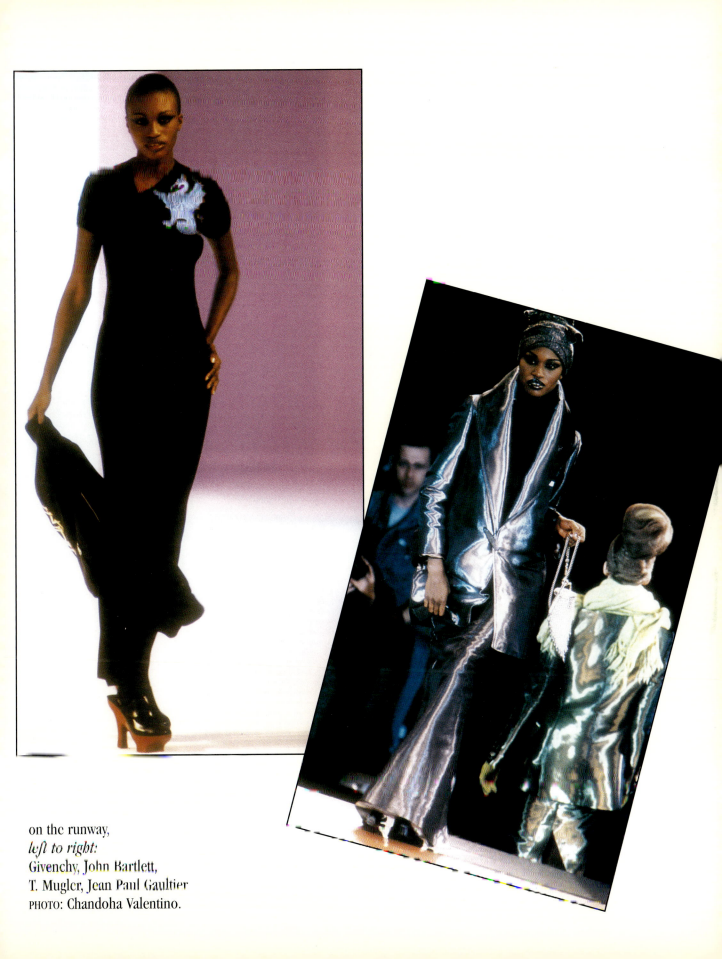

on the runway,
left to right:
Givenchy, John Bartlett,
T. Mugler, Jean Paul Gaultier
PHOTO: Chandoha Valentino.

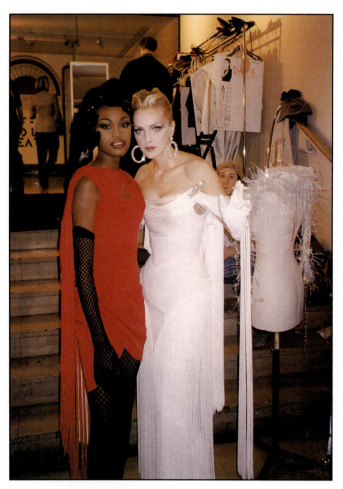

backstage, Theirry Mugler show.

backstage, Givenchy (Alexander
McQueen).

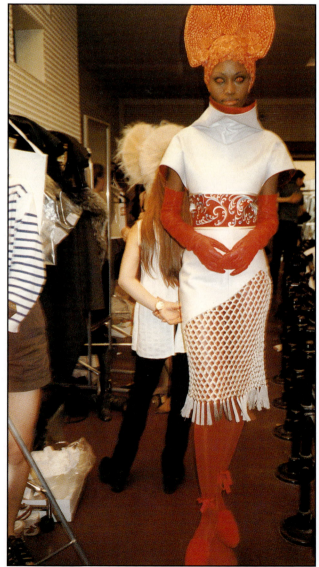

Travel

Travelling is an essential part of modeling. Models must learn to travel light, and to always be prepared, as it is never known when it is time to pack and run for work. I remember on my first few trips to Europe, when I did not necessarily know where my next home will be. I had my entire belongings in two heavy suitcases, which I had to lug with me, from the airport(s) to models' apartments, to train stations, to agencies and to taxis. Luckily, despite all this, I never missed one flight.

It is also imperative for the model to be on top of all legal matters regarding visas for countries that require them, to avoid problems with travelling and work. Not all Immigration Officers will take cash under the counter to let you in their country, as in Mexico, if you have no visa.

When packing a suitcase, it is always wise to include your basic black garments, as they are least likely to be soiled, and can be worn both as a casual outfit or a formal piece.

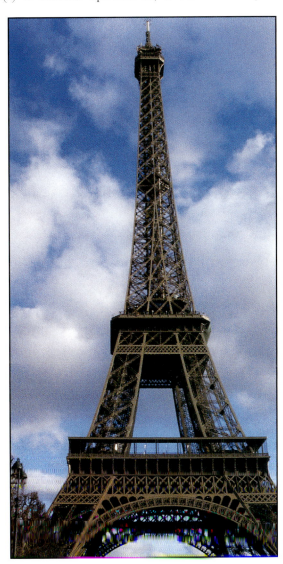

If you are travelling in first class, occasionally asking for a steamed face towel can help in keeping the face hydrated. But if you do not mind travelling in economy, like myself, since the front of the plane is not reaching its destination any faster than the back of it, you may have to devise other ways of hydrating your face. In addition to having a comfortable flight be sure to take a bottle of water, and your facial moisturizers to help in preventing dehydration.

Sometimes it is difficult to rest on flights, but avoid making it a habit to take sleeping tablets as they may become addictive.

Hobbies

As we all know inconsistency is the name of the game in the industry. What is in today is out tomorrow. Sometimes you may go through a period when there is no work for a few weeks or even months. This is the time when you need to focus on other interests, instead of sitting in front of the television all day and getting depressed. When the doldrums hit you, look around and see what you need to know that you do not already know. If there is need to study a subject, do so by going into colleges and applying to do evening classes, or be your own teacher and study at home. Some people go on major shopping sprees in their free time. In Milan, after the shows, models are like ants in the streets getting bargains for their closets. It is some kind of fun, but I never really seem to get pleasure from accumulating too much material things. It seems all a waste to me. After all, I have been given so many clothes from designers, I really see no need to go shopping for more.

I spend my free time writing, painting, reading and taking photographs. Otherwise, you will see me in museums and galleries on the weekends, sometimes going to see performances in the theatres of Broadway, in a movie theatre or at a church. I am always trying to keep myself occupied.

If you are exhausted, going home can be rejuvenating. Yet for me anywhere can be home, once I feel love around me, have a peacefulness within myself and I feel satisfied with my relationship with God. All is well with my soul.

In this profession, where the work schedule is hectic, you should learn to enjoy solitude during slack periods to "recharge your batteries". Then you get to discover yourself more in your free time. Try doing things alone without being in a crowd at all times. I could say you spend so many hours around people in this business, so when you get some time for yourself, it should be pure relief.

"Ms. Rose and great grandchild,
an image I captured
in Top Hill, St. Elizabeth."

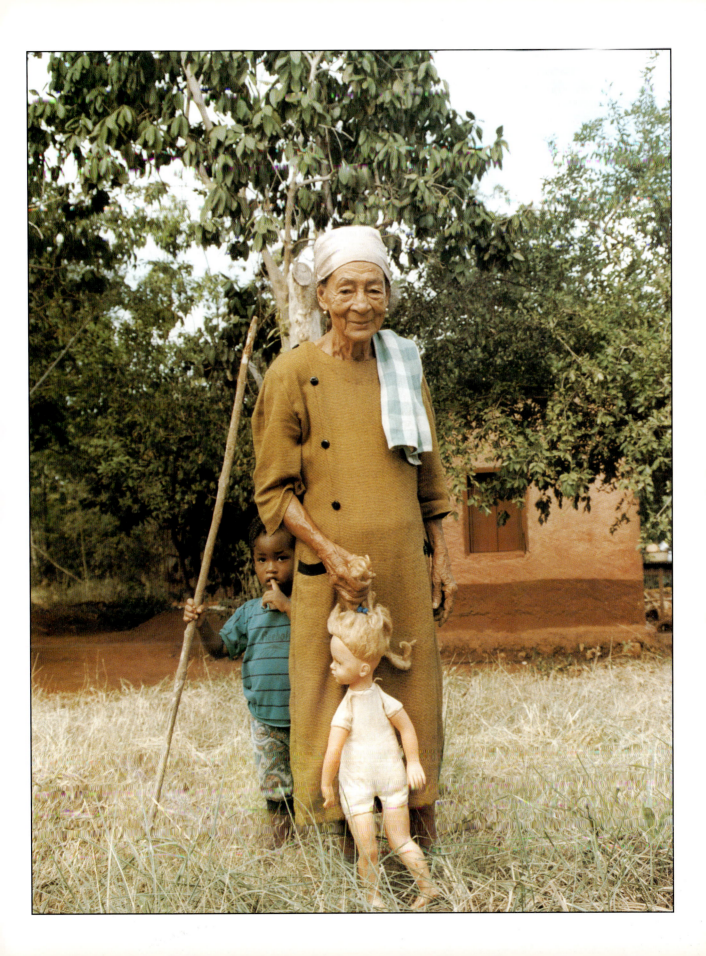

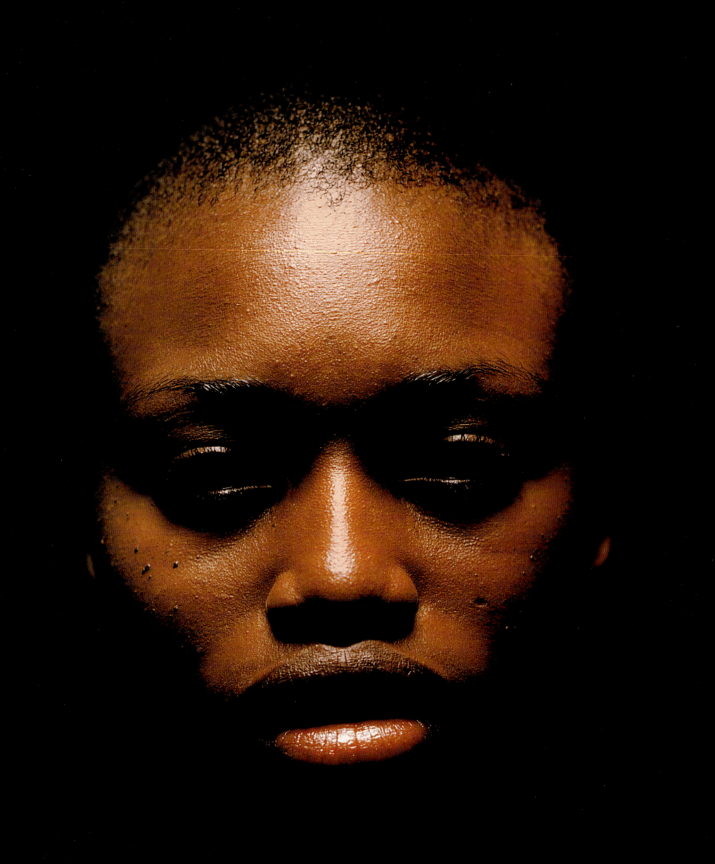

Epilogue

After all my journeys, experiences and achievements, I am happy to write this book, happy to share what the world of fashion is like for me, especially with the people of the Caribbean. Before I ventured out into the world of fashion modelling, I would have welcomed so much a book like this, which sort of gives a guide to what can be expected in this profession, so I could in some way prepare myself. It is great to know that coming from a tiny little dot in the world, anyone armed with capability and determination can achieve the goal that is set for.

Coming from a small island, a gem in the sea, Jamaica, and to go in a white world and Be is to glow.

To come from a tiny village, and to put one foot out into the world and make a foot print, is to glow.

To fight all negatives and turn all negatives into positives is to glow.

You are able to get what you desire, if you try.

Today I still consider myself a free spirit, and have become a child of the universe, living her dreams.

Today I am immensely pleased with all I have accomplished as an international model and am happy to say that all the glitz and glamour has not changed me one bit. I have met beautiful people, worn beautiful clothes and been to beautiful countries, but I still know where the real beauty lies . . . inside you.

Today I live in New York City, in the trendy neighbourhood of Greenwich Village. I ride my bike to the Hudson River; I watch the blazing sun dive in the horizon leaving the red, pink and blue skies behind; I sit and write poetry, I travel the world still working as a model, ever enjoying this job which has so much to offer. It has opened so many doors for me and now I am preparing myself for the future with anticipation of greater heights to climb.

The future for me, Lois, is in the hands of the Great Creator. But my intentions still lie in seeing more, being more, doing more and giving more. Modelling is not a lifetime career, and at times not very fulfilling. After you have seen it and done it, I believe you will start to say, it is time to move on. I have

PHOTO BY **Edward Gorn**

started to work on my second book, where I get the chance to display my love for the arts, using my photography and poetry to portray the sensitivities of the people of Jamaica. I hope that the myriad hues of my country and my people will be faithfully captured. I am also working on other projects, utilizing my experience in fashion, to take it to another level.

Every human being is capable of charting his or her own course in life. Be a captain of your fate and a master of your circumstances. If you visualize positively on all that is good, that good will materialize in your life, and touch others in a most enduring way. Be strong and positive, and always know that *"**one should never be a shadow, but, a glow in the dark**"*.

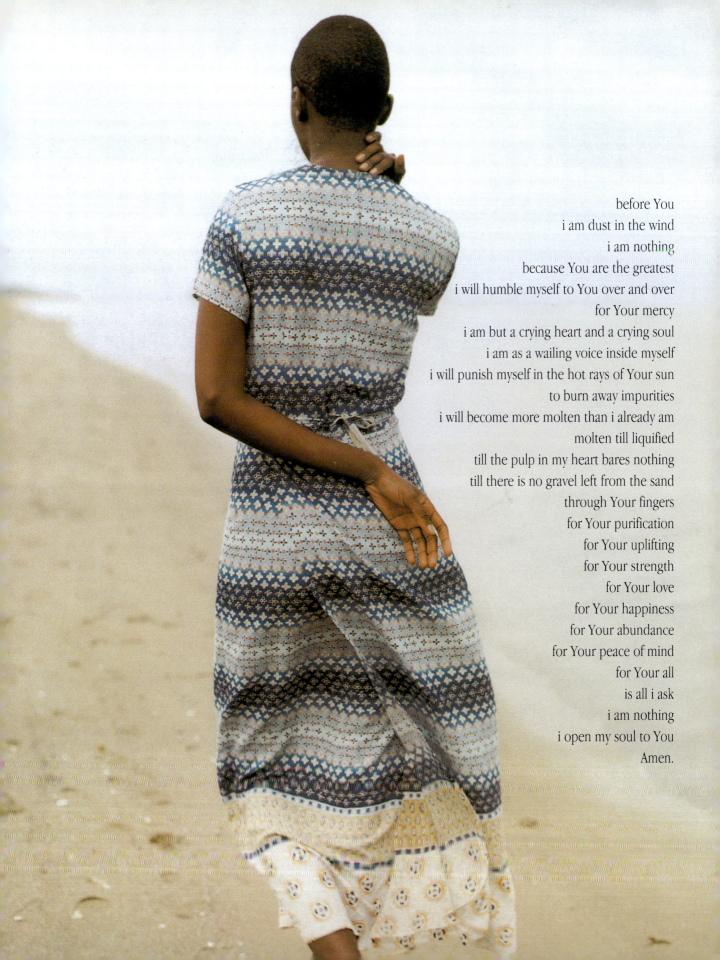

before You
i am dust in the wind
i am nothing
because You are the greatest
i will humble myself to You over and over
for Your mercy
i am but a crying heart and a crying soul
i am as a wailing voice inside myself
i will punish myself in the hot rays of Your sun
to burn away impurities
i will become more molten than i already am
molten till liquified
till the pulp in my heart bares nothing
till there is no gravel left from the sand
through Your fingers
for Your purification
for Your uplifting
for Your strength
for Your love
for Your happiness
for Your abundance
for Your peace of mind
for Your all
is all i ask
i am nothing
i open my soul to You
Amen.

Glossary of Modeling Terms

Manager/Booker

A person in the agency who handles appointments, problems, and bookings.

Booking

A definite job that a client pays for.

Booking Out

Any time a model is unavailable, and her agent notified, so it can be marked on the model's chart that she has booked out.

Call Time

The time a model has to arrive for any appointment or booking.

Cancellation

When a job is no longer booked. All definite bookings regarding compensation, full or partial, to be checked with model's manager.

Castings

A specific appointment, set up with the client for a specific job.

Charts

A time chart, kept by the model's manager or booker, to ensure that the exact whereabout of each model is known.

Checkiing Availability

The time a model usually calls her booker to check her own assignment availability. Important times should be before 9:30 a.m. and between 5:00 p.m. and 6:00 p.m.

Go See

An appointment set up by the model's manager, with a client for a preliminary meeting.

On Hold or Option

Not yet a definite booking, but the client has time reserved for the model.

On Set/Off Set

Different rates for the time spent off-set as opposed to on-set for catalogues and other bookings.

Open Call

When the client requests to see several models at one time.

Overtime

Work exceeding eight hours. Manager(s) should be informed anytime a job runs longer than the original time booked, in order to ensure additional compensation is received by the model. Total time worked on should be reflected in the model's voucher.

Portfolio

A book compiled by the model which has photographs blown up, along with tear sheets, magazine covers and sometimes slides to show clients. Agencies request a minimum of two of these books to send out to clients.

Rate

The amount received for a job. The rate of a booking should be disclosed by the model's manager before the model arrives at a job, so that the proper rate is reflected on the voucher.

Request Only

When the client requests to see only a certain model(s) for a specific job.

Tear Sheets

Actual copies of the work done on a booking, for example, in magazines, newspapes, brochures, posters, etc.

Testing

Photographs taken of a model for her portfolio by various photographers.

Vouchers

A payment form and a contract between a model and the client. Precise information has to be correctly filled in. Triplicates are required: a copy for the client, a copy for the model herself (for retention) and a copy to the accounting department so that billings can be done without delay.

About the Author

Lois Samuels

Born 16 May, 1973, Santa Cruz, St Elizabeth, Jamaica.

Santa Cruz Preparatory School, Jamaica, 1976-1984.

Hampton High School, Jamaica, 1984-1989.

Discovered by Kingsley Cooper of Pulse, Jamaica, 1988.

Jamaica Fashion Model, 1988 and 1991.

Taken Bethann (Hardison) Management, 1993.

Current Agencies— Pulse, Jamaica (Mother Agency), IMG - N.Y., Take2 - London, FAM - Paris., Why Not - Milan, Name - Amsterdam

Modelling Assignments
Advertising

1994 CK One

1994 Anni Kuan Advertising

1995 Samsonite (Amsterdam)

1996 Club Monaco

1996 Jussara Lee Advertising

1996 Isaac Mizrahi, Amtico

1998 Debut Shoe Campaign (Italy)

1998 Oilily Advertising (Amsterdam)

1999 Banana Republic Campaign (U.S.)

1999 Nordstrom Advertising (U.S.)

Magazine Covers

1993 A Magazine

1994 One World

1995 Pride

1995 Essence

1997 German Vogue

Designers

Ralph Rucci, Ralph Lauren, Issey Miyake, Emmanuel Ungaro, Paco Robanne, Armani, Lawrence Steele, Guy Laroche, Moschino, Vivienne Westwood, Christian Dior, Theirry Mugler, Givenchy, Christian Lacroix, Anna Sui, Christophe Lamaire, Yeohlee, Dries von Noten, DKNY, Jussara Lee, Martin Margiela, Jean Paul Gautier, Isaac Mizrahi, Calvin Klein, Marc Jacobs, Tommy Hilfiger, Karl Largerfield, William Calvert . . .

Magazines

Cosmopolitan, Italian, British and German Vogue, French Glamour, Essence, The Face, I-D, Scene, Harpers Bazaar, Paper magazine, Panache, One World, Unfold, Pride, Sky Writings - Air Jamaica, Dutch, Jalouse, Vibe, Interview, Dutch Elle, Donna, Black Elegance, New York Times . . .

Photographers

Peter Lindbergh, Kevin Knight, Cleo Sullivan, Ellen von Unwerth, Steven Meisel, Ruven Afanador, Nick Knight, Albert Watson, Walter Chin, Michael Segal, Marc Baptiste . . .

Other Milestones

Film

Dead Kittens (short film); Director Patricia Murphy: London, 1996

Television

Fashion File VH1, 1994-1998.
The VH1 Awards Show, 1994
The Cosby Show, 1999.